Yes *You* Can!

THE ACHIEVABLE DIET

A Guide to a Positive Mindset and Permanent Weight Loss

by Diana Le Dean

Forward by Dr Naras Lapsys BSc, MSc, PhD, APD

diana.ldb@gmail.com

ISBN-10: 1478207477
EAN-13: 9781478207474
Library of Congress Control Number: 2012915204
CreateSpace Independent Publishing Platform
North Charleston, South Carolina

To my daughter Marina Yasmine and my brother Julian:
Thank you for loving me unconditionally. You are my life.

ACKNOWLEDGMENTS

To Chris, for your love and support.

To my nephews: Paul, Dean, Craig, Mark, George, Izzy, Jack, Emma, Abbey, Mason, Yvette, Stephannie and Holly. Thinking of you gives me the strength to create.

To my brother, Renzo, for loving me.

To Tina and Harry, who always make me feel I can achieve anything I want. Thank you.

To Miranda 'Tiger': this book would have never happened without you. Thank you for your support, determination and care. You go, girl!

To Dr Naras Lapsys. Your knowledge and love of nutrition always excite me.

To Kerry McEvoy. Your 'straight to the point' teaching changed my life.

To Karen, Francesca and Lavinia. Your friendship is invaluable.

To Matthew Perry. Your patience, professionalism and care helped make this book come to life and my dream come true.

TABLE OF CONTENTS

FORWARD

I still clearly remember the first time I met Diana. It was a busy working day, and I had arranged to meet her at my clinic; we were to head out for a quick lunchtime meeting. As I ushered out my last client, I recall looking over at the waiting room chairs and catching a glimpse of a woman who literally glowed. She stood up, stretched out her hand and greeted me with a warm, beaming smile, crystal clear eyes, and an Italian-accented "Pleased to meet you" that instantly transported me to Rome!

Over that lunch, I discovered that Diana's passion and knowledge for nutrition and health nearly surpassed my own. I'm a nutrition researcher with a PhD, and also the principal dietitian of a busy weight-loss and nutrition practice, so that is quite a feat. We discovered that we share the same philosophies when it comes to health, and Diana opened the doors to all her projects, past and present, including this book.

Diana practices what she preaches, and this book is her story. If you want to lose weight or are battling your weight loss demons, this book will get you over the line. You will be inspired, guided, and educated toward making the fundamental changes needed to achieve your ideal weight and health.

As you work your way through each chapter, Diana will become your friend, confidante, coach, and teacher. In this book, she leaves no stone unturned. Her vast knowledge of current nutrition principles, human physiology, psychology, and practical experience all come into play in helping you to achieve and maintain your health and weight goals. Please believe me when tell you that I, too, learned some pearls of wisdom and great ideas that I will certainly be taking back to my own clinic. Every page is filled with knowledge, practical tips, and more importantly, a structured "road map" that leads you through the trials, challenges, and ultimately the triumphs of weight loss.

My life and livelihood is dedicated to nutrition and to the pursuit of better health. If I were to write a book on weight loss, I don't think I would be able to improve on Diana's *Yes, You Can*. For many people, weight loss is not easy, and Diana fully understands and empathizes. This book is her offering to all who are courageous enough to try.

After developing a deep respect and friendship with Diana, and after reading every page of this book, all I can say is I am so glad that I chose the freshest, "cleanest"-tasting sushi restaurant for our fateful first meeting!

Dr. Naras Lapsys, BSc (Hons), MSc, PhDAccredited
Practicing Dietitian, Sydney, Australia

Introduction

DIANA'S STORY, AND WHAT TO EXPECT FROM THIS BOOK

Whoever Writes the Menu Rules Your World

Most of us probably can identify one person who helped us break open the world of food and eating. I lovingly remember two: my French grandmother and my Italian grandmother, both of whom adored me.

I was three years old when my parents divorced. My mother and two brothers stayed in Australia, my father took a job as an engineer in America, and I was enrolled in a wonderful boarding school in Italy. Weekends were spent either with Nonna or Grand-mere. These women, equal in their devotion to their granddaughter, were as opposite as the earth's poles when it came to food.

My French grandmother was very strict with what little she kept in her kitchen, not due to financial reasons but for what I call "French reasons." She simply didn't think food was very important. Why would one spend hours preparing it when there were books to read, ideas to discuss, and walks to take? You ate only because you must. Her dinners usually amounted to little more than soup and some fruit. She claimed that a woman had to look after her beauty; I am sure that today she would replace "beauty" with "health."

And every time I set foot in her house, I heard the "Oh dear, you are getting fat" refrain.

"If you don't want your husband to run away, well, my dear, you simply cannot get fat," she told me, before I could even imagine I might one day *want* to get married. My father used to roll his eyes, give me a complicit wink, and say, "Oh, this is madness!" But he didn't set the menu, and at the end of the day I was still very hungry.

Meanwhile, my Italian *nonna* practically lived in her kitchen. She would cook for two days before my arrival and present heaping plates of meat, fish, potatoes, pasta, and cakes. As soon as I appeared, she would squeeze my face and kiss me all over until I was breathless. Then she would step back, examine me with a practiced eye, and exclaim, "Look at you! You're so skinny I could snap you like a chicken! Soon you will want a boyfriend, and where do you find a boyfriend if you are so skinny?"

My father would roll his eyes and announce, "Oh, this is madness!" (He was a very fair man). And then we would tuck into the enormous dinner Nonna had created. The food was so delicious! I remember thinking that maybe my stomach would actually explode if I tried cramming in another mouthful. Meanwhile, I'd listen to Nonna chatter about what she was going to prepare for the *next* day.

My French grandmother used to say: "Spoil your dinner! Eat an apple or a small piece of bread, or you will get to the table and eat like an animal!" *Like an animal?* I'd think. *All we're having is a bowl of onion soup and peaches for dinner!*

The next weekend, my Italian grandmother would get very upset if she saw me nibbling in the afternoon. "Don't spoil your dinner, for God's sake!" she'd warn me. Then, at dinner, she'd sit back with satisfaction as I went "animal." Nothing gave her more pleasure than watching someone she loved eat. And eat. These visits were sandwiched between weeks at boarding school, where food was simple, healthy, plentiful, and free of culinary drama. I always ate well, and in moderation, because there was no mother or grandmother using food as a weapon of love or frustration. The director of the school was very proud to explain to parents that a physician had created the students' menu. Here, food was nutritionally sound and emotion-free, just what you'd expect from a health professional.

Not surprisingly, from a very young age I understood that the head of a household is in command of the food put on the table. Food is an expression of his or her culture and beliefs about what "good" food really is. I realized that the person in charge of the kitchen wields great power in life.

So as a little girl, I fantasized about what I'd cook when I was old enough to be in charge. *Chicken and cakes daily,* I would think proudly.

For years, I trotted between the two grandmotherly poles, eating just enough or far too much. The scales tipped, you might say, when I was ten and spent a summer with my Italian grandmother. Guess what: Nonna didn't just pull out the stops on weekends. She stuffed me daily. I got fat. When my father arrived for a visit, he took one look and hauled me off to the local doctor.

My father wanted me referred to a weight-loss specialist immediately. But the lovely country doctor took a deep, annoyed breath and said this wasn't necessary.

He turned to me and asked what I had for lunch the day before. I told him: Rice with butter and cheese.

"Good," he said. "Tomorrow have less. Dessert once a week. Whatever you are eating, have less, and ride your bike around or swim wherever. As long as you move and keep moving, you'll be fine." And that was it.

My father was appalled: Who did this lazy quack think he was? But two months later there was no doubt that the doctor's advice was simple *and* wise. I had lost eleven pounds/five kilograms in two months; I remember this precisely because the doctor beamed proudly when I stepped on the scale. There had been no kind of struggle. I ate all the same foods; my Italian grandmother did not have to change her cooking methods or ingredients. But I had adjusted to smaller portion sizes after only few days, and remained faithful to the pledge of dessert once a week. I easily maintained these habits once I returned to school. My French grandmother would have been proud of my restraint, *if* I'd had the nerve to tell her I'd gained the weight!

That was my first lesson in weight loss, the most pleasant and straightforward I ever experienced. I was happy with my slimmed-down figure, especially when a very handsome eleven-year-old boy took quite shine to me at the beginning of the new school term.

Growing Up and Working Out, with a Day of Freedom

Life wasn't just about eating, of course. Almost from day one—literally—I was exposed to the joys and (sometimes) glory of rigorous athletic training.

My brother, who was much older, was the champion of Australian boxing, and he went to the Tokyo Olympics the year I was born. A picture of him once appeared in the newspaper, with tiny little me being coddled on top of his boxing gloves. I learned to toddle in gyms and always looked up my brother both for his achievements and devotion to physical fitness.

So I became a competitive roller skater in my teens. My passion for the sport kept me slim. I worked out for hours on end to refine my skills without thinking about the relationship between exercise and weight. I just was doing what I loved. I competed until the end of high school.

I lost my balance when I was about twenty and began dating a bodybuilder who took part in competitions around the world. He declared that everything I was eating was wrong. Everything. He coached me off the balanced meals that had sustained me for years. Breakfast turned into ten egg whites with boiled spinach, boiled brown rice with olive oil, and a small tank of juice made of carrots, oranges, and whatever fruit was in season. Lunch was always chicken breasts, potatoes, more rice, and a protein bar from the health-food shop. Snack was yogurt with fruit and protein powder. Dinner was yet more rice, with fish, red meat, or chicken. Repeat times six, Monday through Saturday. The only break from the monotony was on the few Sundays when my boyfriend wasn't competing. "All week good and on Sunday free!" he'd declare. On those days we'd indulge in pasta and pastries he loved but almost never touched.

Soon, I was training five times a week on my own. My boyfriend filled bottles of protein powder drinks for me. I got toned like never before, but I'm sure that my French grandmother would have seen me as quite overweight. I was very, very muscular and, secretly, very, very unhappy. For the first time in my life, I felt genuine food cravings. I was always—I mean, *always*—craving the food I was not allowed to eat.

Through the week I dreamed of roasted potatoes with roast beef and dishes of chocolate mousse. Those dreams were downright wicked. I knew actual cheating would have jeopardized my relationship. My boyfriend needed the girl in his life to share his eating and training habits. There could be no discussion about it. I couldn't even to admit my cravings; I was sure he would call me weak and dump me. In love, or at least thinking I was, I tried to keep with his regimen.

As it usually goes in unhappy relationships, the wicked thoughts didn't disappear. They grew ever more vivid. Despite all the calories my bodybuilder's diet contained, it was even more restrictive and monotonous than my French grandmother's. So I constantly dreamed of "naughty" food. I craved it. My virtue didn't stand a chance.

Finally, I bought forbidden food—chocolate—and scarfed it down. Eating it was an orgy of guilt and pleasure. That first piece of chocolate I swallowed on the sly probably tasted as delicious as Eve's apple.

Of course, there wasn't just a single slip. Soon these forbidden trysts were part of my routine. I never cheated on my boyfriend with another man. Cheating on him with food felt just as dangerous, empowering, and depressing.

Meanwhile, I was unhappy about my weight and decided to use the country doctor's method once more. I put less food on my plate and cut my training down from five to two or three times a week. I expected a rebuke, but my boyfriend turned out to be too self-absorbed to notice. The weight I'd put on disappeared. My figure went back to lean and sleek. Of course, eventually even my boyfriend noticed me, and took all the credit!

I made other changes. Instead of spending my money on protein powder, I'd use it to get my hair done. Any guilt I had felt over lying to my boyfriend grew weaker with every positive change I made. Soon, I had my own little program for weight control and exercise that I had begun to share with my girlfriends. Soon after that, I gave the bodybuilder the boot.

Happy to be free again, I was grateful to my beau for one thing: introducing me to the "all week good and on Sundays free: concept. I modified it slightly. One free meal a week seemed like quite enough; a person could pack a lot of living into a multi-course meal! Especially if she was going to Nonna's for Sunday dinner.

Tales from the Dark Diet Jungle

Of course, some of the bad habits from my days of bodybuilding and food cheating endured. I had become a yo-yo dieter, alternating between the healthy "good" foods and the forbidden "bad" ones. I loved the good and the bad for different reasons, and my inability to leave the "bad" alone confused me. Why did I binge? Why would I go into the kitchen and eat chocolate in the middle of the night? Why would I spend a few days eating salad and fruit and then devour a huge chunk of cake from the bakery, even though it was "bad" for me? Why could I not keep my weight under control?

Searching for answers opened me up to some pretty ridiculous solutions. This was the 1980s, and new diet trends popped up every few months. I jumped on just about every one of them and discovered that they shared one critical feature: not one of them broke the yo-yo pattern and ended the nighttime binges that counteracted all the day's good work.

At last, I had an epiphany. I suddenly realized that every diet out there told you why certain foods are bad for you, what *not* to eat, and when *not* to eat it. But none of them addressed the truth about cravings. None had effective means of dealing with them. You just were not supposed to have them, or at least never give in. Restriction and denial were always the key concepts. Think about that: restriction and denial. For a person who genuinely loved food, as I did, that was a pretty miserable prescription.

I was doing better than many people; I was actively researching digestion and nutrition to better understand why cravings strike and what sorts of foods might counteract them. And I had many confused, overweight friends who simply didn't understand why they felt so poorly. To help them, and help myself, I became something of a guinea pig.

Eventually, the lessons of a lifetime began to synthesize. I came to accept that both my grandmothers lived inside of me; opposites though they were, they had to live in harmony through me. There was no denying that food was wonderful, a primary experience that must be embraced. But it was also true that, like all life's passions, I had to control this love or it would control me.

It became clear to me that when I stopped saying no to forbidden foods, the cravings subsided. A free meal helped me to keep good form and controlled portions during the week. I stopped saying no and embraced food on my terms.

At last, I had broken the pattern of yo-yo dieting. I'm still proud of my accomplishment.

I kept talking to my friends about my insights. I continued to emphasize the value of eating a little less and exercising a little more. A lot of unreliable information and crazy fads were obscuring this simple, essential concept. It was no wonder so many of my friends were unhappy.

The Origin of a Method

In the late 1980s I began working as an aerobics instructor in St. Tropez. Done with bodybuilding, I was lean, toned, and no longer muscle-bound. My clients, eager to know how I maintained my form, bombarded me with questions. I'd invite many of them back to my home for advice sessions about eating. I never charged them, since these women were devoted to my aerobics classes at the gym and had helped make my position there secure. But quickly I saw that I was providing my clients with something much, much more than a workout. They were learning how to live healthier lives.

It was a mutually reinforcing pattern: the more I helped others, the more confident I became that the secret to dieting was to love food, not hate it. Of course, that advice was nothing more than a jingle without details and a program to support it. I wanted a regimen for myself as well; the country doctor's advice, after years of extremes, wasn't going to stick unless I knew exactly how I was going to get through each week.

I realized I was one of the few personal trainers who counseled clients about food *and* exercise. At that time, if you wanted to lose weight, likely you'd hire a nutritionist. Either that, or you'd hit the gym. Integrating diet and exercise programs was difficult, because few people knew how to blend the two to fit the needs of each client.

I certainly knew how to help people exercise; between skating, bodybuilding, and aerobics, I'd learned how to sculpt a body and monitor workouts. But my clients also needed clarification about why diets do not work and the long-term benefits of exercise.

I told every client the story of my grandmothers and the country doctor. I interpreted his little message: if you want to lose weight, you eat less of what you *actually like to eat* and make sure you move and exercise more. I told them that smaller portions of food they truly enjoyed would be more satisfying. I insisted they count calories and carb intake faithfully, but not obsessively, to help them make smart dietary choices.

And that was it.

Simple, yes? But, I emphasized that a simple plan and an easy one are not the same thing. At all.

Clients started to get it. They were losing weight, toning up, and enjoying food again.

I was on to something, but there still was a great deal for me to learn about food and the brain's relationship with it. In 1989, I moved to my country of birth, beautiful Australia, to earn certification as a personal trainer and a nutritionist (while enjoying a fit lifestyle and a good income). I enjoyed the exhaustive study of anatomy, physiology, and nutrition, and I deepened my understanding of how diet, exercise, and lifestyle integrate. I often thought about all the diets I'd tried and couldn't believe I'd been taken in.

Most were all about gimmicks. Weight loss never turns on a gimmick. But even the diet plans that were based on sound nutrition didn't work for me or for most people I knew. An overweight person needs to change more than what is put on the dinner plate. All the good nutritional advice in the world is useless if we focus on belly fat and extra chins and neglect the mind. The fundamental outlook on life has to change.

Figuring that out had taken me years. Devising out a program for change became my next obsession.

I knew that if I could take any overweight person into confidence and ask if he or she wanted to become lean, each would answer, "Yes! You know I do! But *how*?" I also knew that a great deal of the advice doled out by personal trainers and nutritionists amounted to "just do it." I'd told some of my own early clients to "just do it," and the misery on their faces was heartrending. Because, of course, if they could just do it...they would! Clearly, they could *not* just do it, no matter how badly they wanted to change.

Who could help them? It had to be someone who understood the ways of binging, yo-yo dieting, the allure of forbidden foods, and how it felt to lack control of what you are eating. Someone who had walked the walk and then walked (and run) free.

I became determined to perfect a system that would help these clients "do it." I expanded my studies to include psychology and counseling. I interviewed people without binging problems or weight-control issues to observe how they thought about and approached food and exercise. Their insights had great relevance to my clients; you will find many of them sprinkled through this book.

Accentuate the Positive: The Key To My Method

Those clients and I worked very hard to push beyond the limited thinking of the diet jungle. "Just do it?" So 1980s. Today we'll begin by saying, "yes, you can."

Saying 'yes' is the essence of my program and a key reason why it's effective: *it's not based on restrictions*. By now, you might have guessed that I'm ambivalent about the word "diet." It smacks of deprivation, of starving yourself, of crazy trends, and of failure. All too often, "diet" really is a synonym for "fad." But let's remember (or discover) that the word "diet" derives from a Greek word that translates as "manner of living." That could mean a great many things; it does *not have to mean* "starve yourself until you're thin" or anything else that seems wrong on the gut level.

I want to reclaim the original definition of "diet"—simply, the food and drink a person *regularly* consumes. When you think of the word in those terms, it's doesn't have to be about deprivation, starving, and craving. It's about balance.

Now, you might suspect that I think all the diet fads are useless, or worse. But really, the problem isn't with the diets themselves, in most cases. All but the kookiest can help a person reach a sustainable weight, *if* that person is in a healthy, sustaining mindset. But we have tons of evidence that most of us aren't. The Western world's obesity epidemic isn't just a physical symptom; it also is evidence of a mindset that resists a sensible attitude towards eating.

Diet "experts" often fail their clients because they gloss over the crux of the matter. "We'll show you how to do it; we'll keep you on track," the weight-loss guru might say. "You can stop scoffing down the cookies; just replace them with chicken and veggies."

Does this work for most people? Of course it doesn't. This shallow thinking doesn't deal with *why* those cookies are so attractive or *how* to stop eating the cookies.

My program will teach you about the how and the why through a system of steps that increase your food knowledge and awareness. Yes, since part of your goal is to lose weight, we can still call this process a "diet." But that's just the beginning. You'll learn about food and exercise. You'll also learn (or relearn) a great deal about yourself. In this program you will:

* *Identify what kind of diet personality you are.* Defining your mental strengths and weaknesses will make you more aware of your eating patterns and triggers.

* *Understand how your body works.* I'll explain the relevant physiology in a very easy-to-understand and enjoyable way. This is the only book you'll need to understand how your body uses food.

* *Increase your nutritional IQ.* You'll learn the about the essential building blocks of food and avoid many weight problems simply by making smarter food choices each day.

* *Become especially aware of the dangers of sugar.*

* *Become mindful of what you're really eating and drinking.* You'll cut down on mindless and emotional eating that happens whether you're hungry or not.

* *Eat the foods you like in proper proportion, based on Green, Yellow and Red lists.*

* *Have a daily weigh-in and find your common weight denominator.* You'll learn not to trust individual numbers and place your faith in averages.

* *Count calories and carb intake without being obsessed.*

* *Incorporate more exercise into your daily life, hitting a gym only if you enjoy it.*

* *Learn that you can lose weight no matter what your age.*

* Accept that weight loss is a process—you go from A to Z. You won't be afraid to let it take all the time necessary. This isn't about dropping thirty pounds in thirty days. It's about dropping thirty pounds for life.

It's important to remember that my methods are based as much on experience with individual clients as they are on what I have learned through research. For instance, I strongly emphasize nutritional counseling because, despite the daily barrage of information about food, few of my clients actually understand even the basic concepts of nutrition. They almost always are shocked to find out that what they thought were healthy choices actually are calorie dense and nutritionally deficient, much more so than what they really want to eat.

I'll never forget Angela, who told me that her favorite food was pineapple. Did she eat it regularly for breakfast, I asked? No. She assumed it was nothing but sugar *just because she liked it*, and that if she liked it must be naughty food! I encouraged her to replace unhealthy choices (they included eating no breakfast at all) with the pineapple she really wanted. That change was essential to her steady weight loss.

You see, the ultimate goal of my program is for you to be happy *and* healthy—happy and comfortable in your own skin, with a healthy body and the energy to match.

Some say that I'm claiming all people can be chubby and happy. But that's not my philosophy at all. You *can* be beautiful if you're chubby; if you believe you're beautiful then you are! But if you're seven pounds/three kilograms over your ideal weight and you feel awful about yourself, you'll never be happy until the pounds are gone.

The point is this: my program is not about size. It's about being comfortable with and loving your own body. No matter what dress size you aspire to wear, we will get you there. And you'll be healthier than you were before you began the journey.

I've written this book as the next-best substitute for me being in the room with you. I'll show you how to manage your relationship to food. You'll turn the tables and allow your love of certain foods to become healthy and open, and under *your* control. You'll say good-bye to secret, forbidden, "bad" foods: Play out that drama somewhere else!

It's essential that you realize that you have the power to enact these changes. Often, during the course of our conversations, my clients tell me what is best for them before I do. Some figure out solutions to the issues we've been discussing on their own. Once you've read this book carefully, you can do the same.

The wisdom of an Italian grandmother, a French grandmother, an athletic brother, a country doctor, and many other people in my life has produced this book. They all helped me raise my IQ in nutrition, fitness, health, and beauty; now it's my turn to help you achieve through small, important steps. You'll soon be able to change your nutritional program any time you want by making smart food substitutions. You will also be able to enjoy your favorite fatty or sugary foods at least once a week. You will feel empowered and in control, and who knows what else might happen once you're secure in that mindset.

So read on. Learning a new way of life begins with the first step.

Chapter One

A BEGINS THE ALPHABET

L et's get started!

Now, I don't mean we're starting with the main course of the program. It's important to begin with a small taste of the concepts involved, and to savor a small measure of early success. So take a seat, and let's talk about an important human truth.

Everyone Has Blind Spots

This is a simple fact. *We all have blind spots.* It's a big world out there (and in here), and some of it is frightening. Better not to see it, or so we think.

Ignoring the reality of the situation and allowing your actions to be dictated by love, concern, or natural prejudice creates a blind spot. The universal existence of blind spots binds us together; how we *deal* with them sets us apart, especially when we confront a challenge like weight loss.

To deal with yours, learn to spot the giveaway clues. A psychological blind spot often is covered by that "*no-no-no*" response you utter, almost unthinkingly, when someone hits a nerve by saying something you don't want to hear. "No-no-no": it's defensiveness, a desire to remain blind to the truth.

If you're a parent, there might be a blind spot at work even when it comes to your kids. I've counseled mothers who desperately wanted to help their daughters to lose weight. When I calmly asked, "How do you expect to help your daughter to lose weight if your kitchen is stuffed with sugar of every kind: cookies, cakes, snacks, and chips?" the answer usually was: "Oh well, well, er, I just buy those things so she can have one or two when she feels like it." Seeing things clearly? I don't think so.

For these mothers, allowing "a few" cookies expresses love. They don't see that they're sabotaging their daughters' efforts to lose weight.

When there is food in our kitchen, we eat it. That's why we buy it in the first place. Mothers who buy cookies for their daughters and expect them to eat one or two are blinding themselves to human nature. If they believe that their overweight daughters have enough self-control to eat one or two cookies from the box, great. Oh, and why not give the girls the family credit cards, too?

Of course, most mothers would refuse to give their young children credit cards because they accept that the kids aren't yet ready to control their spending. They shouldn't be given free reign in the kitchen, either. But the obesity statistics don't lie: many children are given freedom with food they aren't ready to handle.

Obviously, you should apply this logic to your own life. Stop saying that you'll savor that sugary/salty food you love in small, controlled portions. Just don't buy it.

You know how difficult it will be to resist eating it all, quickly. Why put yourself through such torture? Let me explain this in a different way: DON' T BUY IT!

If you've already detected a blind spot in your food view, maybe you read that paragraph and took action. Maybe you ran to the kitchen and threw away all the food you know will make you fat. Great. You're ahead of the game.

But don't despair if you're still sitting. You know more than you think. You don't need me to tell you what the dangerous foods are: ice cream, cookies, cakes, chips, those packages of dry, sugar-coated fruits, etc. Beyond small doses these foods are not good for you. Yes, you knew that, too. Sugar, salt: no good. That's just common sense.

Take that surprised look off your face, right now! You can't afford to live with this blind spot any longer! *You buy foods that are not good for you and you know which foods they are.*

Maybe you accept this fact, but you don't want to throw that food away because you paid for it, because it's wasteful, etc. You're still in the blind spot. Buying food you know to be unhealthy is evidence of an unthinking cycle that you must end. Take aggressive action. This one time, the last time, make a statement: throw it out!

Your kitchen must be purged of unhealthy food, and you need a small accomplishment that marks the beginning of your transformation and instills a little pride in you.

So make this gesture and throw out the dangerous food in your kitchen. You'll make room for organic cooking books, your Vogue magazine collection, and maybe a plant or two. Clear space for new food and energy.

Still need some help? Let's go together. Take a big bag and remove all the high-calorie, unhealthy food from your fridge and all the cupboards in your kitchen. Yes, I hear you: "No, not my chocolates!" Later on, you *will* be able to eat your favorite chocolate, a piece of cake, and some chips, regularly! I don't believe in deprivation, but I also don't believe in stuffing your kitchen with enough sugar to sustain a rugby team for a month.

So whether it's salty chips, chocolate, cookies, frozen pizzas, or instant mashed potatoes, today it's got to go in that big bag. We'll go into the details of this food's low nutritional value in chapter two. The goal here is to break the habit of grabbing a cookie—or five—whenever the urge strikes. When we're done, there should still be plenty of good food left. Nobody ever gets fat from eating too much broccoli or tuna.

When the sweep is done, congratulate yourself. I mean it. You've taken the important first step that should have exposed at least one blind spot about food and your diet. Chances are, if you have been overweight for some time, there are spots that affect your relationships with people and food. Today, you learned that awareness expands whenever you choose to break down your psychological defenses.

Little Steps Count

Now you have feng-shuied your kitchen, and it is nice and clean. Umm, you think. Is this going to be one of *those* diets? Strict, forbidding, focused on bad behavior?

Cheer up. We're going grocery shopping. Once all that unhealthy food is in the trash, you need to start making some substitutions.

What's your favorite flavor of ice cream, your favorite brand of cookies, or the chips that taste best? Next time you shop, don't buy that favorite. Buy a flavor or brand you don't fancy as much. You love chocolate ice cream but are lukewarm on strawberry? Guess what? You should buy strawberry ice cream. You love salami-and-cheese pizza? Buy a vegetarian, no-cheese option.

Chances are, once you're home it's going to take you much longer to polish off this substitute. Or, in the case of the pizza, you've got a healthier option than your old favorite. After your grand sweep through the kitchen, this will seem like a small, even insignificant step. But it's the small tricks that will help you gain momentum in my program. And they will help you to start shedding weight.

Before you even enter a supermarket, I can throw in another little tip: don't spend five minutes jockeying for a parking space close to the entrance. Park farther out and walk a few steps. When you get home, don't take the elevator or if you have none, stop complaining about walking up four flights. Every step you take is movement, and every movement counts toward your ultimate goal.

And don't be blind to habits that help you gain the weight. If you can't pass the bakery without buying a croissant or a doughnut—yes, you got it—change routes! Save some money! Keep building up the small steps!

I know, I've heard it many times: You want to lose all your weight *now*! *Fast*! I understand. But *fast! now!* is the tempo of yo-yo dieting. If you're serious about keeping off the weight you lose, you'll start by making a string of small, achievable changes. So exchange your favorite dessert for a blander one. Park a little further from the market and walk (or walk *all* the way, if that's feasible). Walk around the bakery, not into it.

Blind and Inactive

Let's talk about exercise. Clients often tell me, *"No-no-no, I can't do physical activities. I have no time; seriously I have no time."* No-no-no: say hello to another blind spot!

Those clients have the time, and so do you. True, that time needs to be set aside, but you're capable of planning. You know there is someone out there with a schedule even crazier than yours who makes time to exercise every single day. If you're "too busy" to exercise, you are just languishing in a blind spot.

Or you may insist that the exercise habit is too expensive. OK, I won't argue (although I probably could). So walk around the park, vacuum the house, or clean the car—just move. Moving your body means burning calories, and burning calories means losing weight. You don't need a treadmill at home or in gym; your exercise can be completely free. If you're still sitting down, look closer. Find that blind spot! There is no reason you cannot find something to do, right now that will burn a few more calories.

Beginner steps? Yes, they are. But recognize how much healthier your life can become if you cut out eating highly caloric foods just by substituting one food for another or changing your morning route to work. Count the number of exercise minutes you could log if you took a walk during your lunch break instead of sitting at your desk. Life does not have to be so complicated. We make it complicated.

Once you've got a few of these simple but effective, small steps in your routine, keep at them. And while you're losing a little weight, let's move onward.

The A-to-Z Process

My A-to-Z weight-loss method was in part inspired by the work of Dr. Stephanie Burns, author of *Great Lies We Live By*. Dr. Burns argues that you can train yourself to learn most anything *if* you understand that there is process in everything you do, and can endure beyond a tipping point that occurs about six or seven weeks after you've started. This is when the excitement and novelty of your new endeavor begin to wear off, and the repetition often becomes boring and difficult. It gets harder and harder to keep on going, and many of us, once enthusiasts for a new skill or way of living, simply give up.

Losing weight is a process. You must accept that changing eating habits of a lifetime will entail some difficulty. Some of the changes may be boring and not to your liking. A primary challenge is developing a new resistance, saying no to pleasures you've indulged time and again.

But if you can envision this build-up of resistance as a process within a process, each battle with a craving for bad food becomes part of the process, too. Understanding and valuing this expansion is the key to feeling empowerment with each small accomplishment, to feeling that yes, you can.

As saying no to fattening foods becomes less a struggle and more routine, you may well find that the same process-developing techniques will help you to say no to other conditions in your life that make you unhappy and, quite likely, played a role in your weight gain.

A is your starting point. Z will be your optimal state of mind and a happy, healthy, and consistent weight.

Some people practically fly from A to Z. Others will master A and B and stay stuck on C for a while, where they encounter some stubborn blind spots and eating habits. They may just find it terribly difficult to switch from French fries to baked potatoes. These people are just as eager to lose weight as anyone else, and when they encounter resistance early, they quite understandably feel scared and worry that they're messing up or failing. But they aren't. They're simply fighting through a tough patch of their journey.

Let's imagine your weight-loss goal in part requires a switch from french fries (A) to baked potatoes with butter (B) to baked potatoes with less butter (C) and ending with baked potatoes with a *sprinkle* of cheese (D). Some people will make that switch in a day, cutting out the intermediary steps. That's great. But it's pointless to despair if it's a struggle simply to stop eating French fries.

Think of it this way. Imagine you're walking to work on a bitter, snowy day. You slip on the ice and fall down. What do you do? You get up, hope that not a lot of people saw you, pull your skirt down, and keep on going. You don't get up and go home! You don't sit on the ground freezing, either.

So when you cave in to the urge to eat the french fries, don't beat yourself up! Just move on, stay calm, and try to remain on track for the rest of the day. And most all, make sure you *enjoy* the french fries. Own the activity. My method is about enhancing joy, not outlawing it!

You might find it helpful to map out the entirety of the A-to-Z weight-loss plan before you start. While every person's plan is unique, below is an outline that is typical for motivated beginners:

A — You read my book and understand the concepts within it.

B — You start to understand what your blind spots are and work to detect them.

C — You score a symbolic, opening victory by ridding your kitchen of the foods you know are not healthy.

D — You shop for less-attractive substitutions. (chapter two will provide further details on making smart substitutions)

E — You decide what your personal ideal weight is.

F — You get a complete checkup from your doctor to ensure there are no underlying health issues.

G — You slowly detox from sugar. (Read all about this in chapter two.)

H — You feel more in control of what you eat. You are more mindful of your emotional eating and discover new ways of dealing with it.

I — You master the fundamentals of weight loss, including portion control, exercise, regular weigh-ins, and allotted times to indulge.

J — You embrace the concept of Red Light, Orange Light and Green Light foods, as outlined in chapter six.

K — You flesh out your grocery list and your favorite food list.

L — You realize how many different, exciting kinds of food there are with less calories and better nutritional value that you can easily substitute for fatty or sugary food. Every week you make small changes to your grocery list to incorporate Green Light Foods.

By the time you've reached L, your lifestyle will have changed dramatically. You will be losing weight without diet trauma; you'll be learning steadily about food and nutrition; ice cream (or chocolate or chips) happily will still on the menu, at the right time in the right portion.

M — Like a marathoner hitting stride, you begin to feel deeply empowered and in command of your process. You are slimming down noticeably, substituting for yet more foods and increasing your activity. There's likely to be some slips even at this point, in the guise of chocolate cake or French fries, but they no longer will threaten your momentum.

N — You begin to branch out physically, trying new activities with the energy that your improved nutrition and attitude deliver.

O — Now you know what healthy food you like to eat, what exercise you like, and you miss it if you don't work out.

P — You become acutely aware of hunger and become skilled at differentiating between a mindless desire to eat and a genuine hunger pang.

Q — Adequate servings of water enable your good nutrition and overall health.

R — You know how to savor your food, and you're becoming even more adventurous and health conscious while you plan your free weekly meals.

S — You become adept at avoiding food cravings. You do not understand how you could have eaten the way you did before!

T — You start to become aware of sabotage: the people in your life and conditions that directly contributed to your unhealthy past tendencies.

U — You accept responsibility for the conditions that you didn't change earlier and distinguish the people who sabotaged out of love versus those who just sabotaged.

V — You find effective means to counteract sabotage that embraces your friends and neutralizes your enemies. (You'll know them when you see them!)

W — You aspire to juggle it all—family, friends, and work—while integrating your new approach to food and fitness with all parts of your life. Some days are better than others, but overall quality is on the upswing.

X — You compile more information about how to maintain your ideal body through stages in life still to come.

Y — You learn how to communicate with your family and incorporate your new food attitudes into communal life.

Z — You are at your ideal weight, or very near it. You are beginning to apply the same techniques you used to lose weight successfully in other areas in your life: relationships, your career, and your finances.

This road map should show you that losing weight is about much more than knowing what a calorie is and hitting a gym. Food is central to our lives, so weight loss is a *lifestyle* change. It will touch almost every other part of your existence.

Those who follow my program all the way to Z will be treating their bodies like temples. Yes, you can do it, too. In order to get there, though, you need to keep moving, like the determined turtle in its race against the hare.

Lose the Guilt

What the majority of people call "failure," I call part of a process. If you can learn to accept your setbacks as normal functions of human nature, you can stop the guilt. Before you embark on your own A-to-Z journey, factor in the stumbles. Expect them; deal with them as they occur, and move on.

Think of any other process you've mastered in your life. Initially, you probably took two steps back for every step forward, but before you knew it, that ratio was reversed. Eventually, those backward steps became rarities. It will be the same with my approach to weight loss.

Besides, we are not always perfect partners, mothers, lovers, or employees, either! It is absolutely predictable as well as acceptable that some months you're going to lose five pounds/two kilograms and the next month you're going to plateau, or even gain a couple of pounds, even though you're eating less. Of course, you'll want an explanation; you'll want to know what you "did wrong." But you won't be doing *anything* wrong. This is just how weight loss works.

And recognize that there is no real "finish line." Your ideal weight is an admirable goal to aspire to, but the greater goal is to try to enjoy the process, all the way from A to Z. There is a victory—or several—to be savored at every letter point. Becoming healthier and happier should be like reading a delightful story with plot twists, sudden character development, and plenty of surprises. It's like a book that you can reread over and over again, each time discovering something new.

It's my hope that you will return to *this* book repeatedly for encouragement and support, consulting it for reminders about the various steps in your personal process. It should be a companion to you, a friend, a shoulder to cry on, a resource when you need to rejuvenate your will power.

Health and Happiness: Set the Terms

"So who is at a healthy weight?" you may ask.

The variety of weight-loss goals and motivations is almost endless. Some of us are within our normal weight range but just want to shed a few pounds we don't need, for a special event perhaps or just to attain a sleeker, shapelier look. Women planning pregnancies ask me for their ideal nine-month nutrition and exercise regimens. Maybe you are combating serious medical problems or fear that you soon will be. Since I'm something of a human Google of information about body sculpting and exercise, I've helped plenty of people who actually wanted to *gain* some weight—muscle weight—without getting too bulky.

Of course, every one of us has a distinct, precise definition of what a "healthy" body is, or should be. But there are some general characteristics that I apply to every person who is at a healthy weight.

By my definition, if you're a "healthy" person, your body is working the way it's meant to work. All of your vital signs are normal for your age; your weight is appropriate for your height; you have strong, toned muscles; your skin (which is your body's largest organ) is vibrant and supple; and you are aerobically fit, meaning that you can perform sustained cardiovascular exercise without stress.

But most important of all, you are mentally fit and in a good place emotionally. There are countless people who become unbelievably miserable while trying to keep their weight under control. Inevitably, their physical health begins to suffer as well. Balance in diet and bodily function is lost easily when you're upset; if you're unhappy while you're slimming down, it will be hard to stick to any program. Trust me when I say that losing weight not only *can* be a pleasant and comfortable experience, it should be if it's to have long-term success!

Most of us begin with unrealistic goals for how much weight we want to lose and, especially, how quickly we want to lose it. That's a recipe for unhappiness. You will need to get your expectations in sync with gradual physiological change. People who tell me they want to lose fifteen pounds/seven kilograms in a month have been influenced by fad-diet claims. Certainly they can lose that much eventually, but no balanced approach to weight loss delivers those kinds of instant returns.

Once you have a reasonable goal in mind, you must get all the medical information you need. Before you adopt my plan in earnest, you should have a complete medical checkup, with comprehensive blood tests, to make sure there are no ongoing or underlying health problems. You should never undertake this program—or any other change to your diet and exercise routines—without the basic facts about your body's primary systems.

Some people begin my program with serious medical diagnoses, diabetes being perhaps the most common. Many more think they are healthier than they are. I've met many people, especially in America, who have been told by their physicians that they're "fit fat," meaning that their blood pressure, vital signs, and blood work are normal, although their weight is high. It's true that some overweight people are, indeed, healthy, especially if they work out regularly and have strong bones and muscles. But many who hear those magic "fit fat" words think they have carte blanche to eat whatever they want and not exercise. Meanwhile, minor complaints they have today could become serious problems later on. "Fit fat" might sound like a happy condition, but for some clients it covers up yet another blind spot.

That said, not everyone needs to hit their lowest physiologically beneficial weight to feel they've really accomplished something. In my program, optimal health and happiness do not have to be synonymous.

As one example, my client Cynthia was very heavy. When we first talked, it was clear to me that she should lose about thirty pounds/fourteen kilograms in order to be at a normal weight for her height, although her doctor's report showed me that she was in decent health.

"What brings you here today?" I asked.

"I'm not happy," she replied.

"OK, you're not happy, that's a big thing. What do you think would make you happy?"

"Well, I'd like to lose six kilograms (thirteen pounds)."

I said that was a smart goal for Cynthia to set. Partly, this was tactical. I'm quite sure that if I'd responded, "Well, I think you should really aim for fourteen kilos," Cynthia would have gotten a negative message. What's the point in making a client feel terrible just at the point she's attempting to make a change?

But there was also a greater consideration. Maybe Cynthia needed to lose thirty pounds/fourteen kilograms in a strict, clinical sense. But if a loss of fourteen pounds/six kilograms left her in better health and at optimum happiness, that made it a smarter goal.

Embrace the Process

Remember that gaining your extra weight was a process, too. It took you quite a lot of time—likely years—to put it on; you have to accept that it will take plenty of time to remove it!

Your positive attitude during the process will be as critical halfway through as it is during the first small steps. Research has shown that those who successfully achieved their weight-loss goal aren't overly analytical; they focus on just getting things done and how they'll feel once the tasks are complete. If you choose power walking as a new exercise option, you won't help your cause by dwelling on how exhausting the walk will be or whether people will know what you're up to. Far better to think about how gratifying the rest of the day will be with that walk completed and out of the way.

Never underestimate the value of repetition. Repeating what you do, at least five times, is a key component of helping you change a habit.

You must also see the negative effects of envy. It's hard not to feel envious when you see someone who appears to have an incredibly perfect body. *I want to look like that,* you think. *I want to look like that right now.* We've all been there.

But you should practice a new attitude. If you see some beautifully toned creature, ask yourself how he or she maintains that fine form. What's his exercise routine like? What and how much does she eat? What did she look like two years ago? What does he find most difficult about keeping up a healthy routine? What routine works best for her?

I can assure you that very few people have fantastic figures without plenty of work and dedication. Don't waste time envying them. Learn about them instead.

I remember when I went skiing for the first time. I watched glorious women ski with grace and confidence that astounded me. How did they move so effortlessly, as if the skis were extensions of their bodies? Eventually I realized that on their first days, they had been no more competent that I was. They had started on the same bunny slope, fallen countless times, then picked right back up and kept trying.

Accept the challenge your new process presents, and you've made a huge step forward. Recognize that you will not achieve your ideal weight today or tomorrow. With patience and perseverance, though, you *will* achieve it, and probably sooner than you think. Keep working, and your "perfect body" will be whizzing down the bunny slope and others will envy *you*.

Summary

- *Recognizing your blind spots is a powerful tool for starting your weight loss.*

- *Remove unhealthy foods from your kitchen and use the storage for something else.*

- *Substitute your favorite unhealthy foods for your "second favorite" healthy foods.*

- *Weight loss is a process from A to Z. Stay calm and carry on.*

Chapter Two

DETOX FROM SUGAR

Sugar's Stealthy Assault

Have you ever tried to cut sugar out of your diet? Did you start by phasing out all the sweet stuff, the cookies, candy, colas, and other usual suspects? How long did the prohibition last? Did you feel irritable while you were denying yourself sugar and guilty when you fell back into old habits?

If you're reading this book with the intent of controlling your weight, I have to deliver some sobering news: more than likely, you are addicted to sugar. Probably you have been for years.

I don't use the word "addicted" lightly. Giving up all refined and unrefined sugars is as difficult as giving up nicotine, alcohol, or hard drugs, if not more so. The body does not like giving up fuel it has come to depend on, no matter how poisonous that fuel really is. The fact is that sugar, that fine white powder you slip into your morning coffee, is just as addictive as cocaine.

Sugar is perfectly legal, and it doesn't give you lung cancer. But it, too, can wreak havoc on your body by contributing to obesity and a host of related medical woes: diabetes, heart disease, arthritis, and yes, cancer. Sugar is sweet, too, so it's difficult to believe that it contributes to so much physical misery. But it does. Know sugar for what it is: an addictive substance that, in the end, can kill you, just like drugs with more sinister reputations.

And of course, sugar is pushed right out in the open market. It's just about everywhere in our society. Forces are in place to encourage your addiction and even deepen it. The food industries of many countries have worked very hard to build up our dependency on their products, and in large part they've succeeded thanks to sugar.

I'm starting this chapter out in a gloomy tone because it's important that you realize the leading role that sugar has played in perpetuating your above-healthy weight. I've told many clients over the years that they must embark on a sugar detoxification if they hope to change their eating habits and lose weight they don't want.

But there is good news, too. Through education, a detailed process, and a lot of hard work, many of those clients went on to successfully wean themselves from sugar. Some gave it up and will never go back. Many, though, have learned how to incorporate sugar into a healthy diet through control and awareness. Yes, you can do the same. First, though, you need some context.

Nations of Sugar Abusers

A person eating the typical Westernized diet consumes about 150 pounds, or 68 kilograms, of sugar every year. A woman of average size eats her own weight—or even more—in sugar every year. Daily, that average person eats about thirty-one teaspoons (about 124 grams) of sugar. At sixteen calories per teaspoon, that's five hundred extra calories.

Since sugar and sugar substitutes have crept into just about every packaged food in the first world, its influence continues to increase. When one food manufacturer adds sugar to a product and finds it sells better, competitors follow the lead. The average man is now getting about 15 percent of his total daily calories from sugar, the average woman about 12 percent. That's a lot more than nutritionists recommend; the American Heart Association, for instance, strongly recommends getting no more than 5 percent of your total daily calories from sugar. If you're eating two thousand calories a day, that means no more than one hundred calories, or about twenty-four grams, from added sugar. (The natural sugar in fresh fruit and dairy products such as milk doesn't count). That amounts to a recommendation of just *six* teaspoons of sugar per day.

So do the math: thirty-one teaspoons of sugar daily with a recommendation of six. The average person is consuming *five times* more sugar than he or she should be.

You're gaining weight? No wonder. You're almost certainly struggling with a sweet addiction.

How does the addiction occur? The explanation involves physiology, emotion, and the environment in which we live. All provide powerful stimuli that make our natural attraction to sugar overpowering.

The sweet taste of sugar stimulates your brain to produce endorphins, your body's natural feel-good chemical. It's exactly the same pathway activated by opiate drugs and nicotine. If you've ever tried to quit smoking, you know how difficult it is to overcome your body's desire for its addictive chemicals.

Sweet foods taste good, of course, but what really hooks us is the way sugar makes us feel. If we're tired and hungry, a candy bar or cookies gives us an energy lift. Desiring the taste of sweetness is also a very deep part of our psychological makeup. Mother's milk, the first taste we encounter, is sweet. In fact, newborn babies can't taste any flavors except sweet. As children, we're often rewarded or comforted with sweets such as candy or cookies, and that comfort lasts into adulthood. When we're upset, sad, lonesome, or feeling neglected or unloved, sugary foods soothe us in a way that friends and family can't or won't.

We feel hunger and emotion in the same place, a big hole between the chest and the hips. Sugar can fill that hole and act like a sedative, at least for a little while.

A few days before I know my husband will be leaving for a weeks-long business trip, I become anxious about the separation. I go crazy for sugar; it's a quick-and-dirty means to soothe my anxiety. It's also a holdover from my childhood. My father would give me chocolate before *he* left on business trips. We never really outgrow the emotions that surround sweet foods.

Meanwhile, food manufacturers have become adept at making products infused with artificial sweeteners appear healthier than they are. And millions of us are taken in. But sugar is sugar, no matter what it's called, and these foods have plenty of calories—and sometimes just as many as versions made with ordinary sucrose (table sugar) or that cheap substitute, high-fructose corn syrup. Packaging can be very deceptive; often a container proclaims that the food inside has no added sugar, but that food is naturally high in sugar—dried fruit is a good example.

On top of that, sugary foods are so widespread today that they're almost impossible to avoid. The workplace often is a sugar minefield. Go to a staff meeting, and doughnuts and cookies are often right next to the coffee; the leftovers end up in the break room. The receptionist has a candy dish on her desk. And how can you refuse a piece of cake at an office birthday party? If the boss gives you a hard time for missing a deadline or coming in late, it's easy to soothe yourself with sugar so you can get back to work.

The supermarket is a giant sugar warehouse. Shelf after shelf, aisle after aisle is nothing but sugar in various forms: candy, cookies, soft drinks, juices, breakfast cereals, energy bars. It's added to almost every packaged food, even salad dressing and savory sauces. "Healthy" options, such as apple juice, yogurt, and dried fruit, often are enhanced with sugar. Sugar even makes it into spaghetti sauce and pizza.

The leading source of added sugar in the typical Western diet is beverages. A typical can of cola, for instance, has about ten teaspoons—or forty or more grams—of sugar. But other beverages do their part, too. Fruit "juices" are heavily sweetened with high-fructose corn syrup; sports and energy drinks often are nothing but sweetened water and chemicals; supposedly healthy milk drinks can pack nearly thirty grams of sugar.

In America, soft drinks account for more diet calories, about 9 percent of daily total, than any other substance. Sweetened fruit juices are very popular in France and Italy, where it is very hard to find natural juice without added sugar. In Australia, 100 percent fruit juice can be found in most supermarkets, but it's often sold in two-liter bottles. You end up drinking a lot of it just to finish the bottle, which means more extra calories than you might realize.

It's easy to see why sugar-enhanced foods are playing a major role in expanding the world's waistline. Meanwhile, sugar has *no* lasting nutritional value other than calories—it has no fiber, no vitamins, no minerals. All it adds to the food is additional sweetness in the form of empty calories.

But sugar's influence over our physiology and minds can't be underestimated. You know, of course, that too much sugar is bad for you; and you probably want to cut back, but you can't. When you don't get your sugar fix, you feel anxious and irritable, driven to find something sweet. When you know sugar is available, it takes up all your attention. Can you concentrate on work knowing there's a chocolate bar in your desk drawer? No, it draws you in like a beacon. You'll probably have to eat it if you want to concentrate.

So before you fall yet again into despair or anger over your inability to stop eating sugar, give yourself a break. The deck has been stacked against you, probably since birth. Sugar addiction has been beneficial to a large chunk of the world's economy, and that won't change anytime soon. If you have become addicted, you've certainly be enabled almost every step of the way.

For your health's sake, though, it's time for you to take action. Fortunately, sugar addiction can be beaten, too. There are no sugar rehab centers (although there probably should be, and I suspect there soon will be), but you can take steps toward detoxification now.

Understanding the Chemical Basics

The fix, the crash, and the need for another fix: it's a cycle well-known to many addicts. We tend to talk about the "sugar crash" in a lighthearted way, as a pseudoscientific means to explain a bad mood or lack of energy. But there's hard science to back up our perceptions.

Sugar has a huge impact on your insulin levels. Insulin is the hormone produced by your pancreas that regulates the amount of glucose (blood sugar) in your bloodstream. When you eat something sweet made from processed carbohydrates, such as white flour mixed with plenty of sugar, your blood sugar jumps way up almost immediately. That triggers your body to release a lot of insulin, which carries some of that extra sugar into your cells to use for energy—and stores the excess as fat.

But when you produce a lot of insulin to clear away a surge of blood sugar, your body can go too far in the other direction. The insulin can carry off so much of your blood sugar that it might dip too low. Within half an hour of eating that sugary food, you crash. You feel tired and cranky, have trouble concentrating, and might even get shaky or nauseous. You get very hungry, because when your blood sugar drops too low, your body thinks you need what? More sugar, to jump back up to normal levels! So you eat more sugar and start the cycle all over again. For people with onset or full-blown diabetes, the swings in your blood sugar are even stronger.

Refined sugar—the white stuff in your sugar bowl—is known chemically as sucrose. Every molecule of sucrose contains one molecule of glucose (the sugar your body uses for energy) linked to one molecule of fructose. So a spoonful of sugar is really half a spoonful of glucose and half a spoonful of fructose (In high-fructose corn syrup, the ratio varies somewhat: a spoonful of this stuff is about 55 percent fructose and 45 percent glucose).

Why this little chemistry lesson? Because it's important to know that your body uses glucose and fructose in different ways. The glucose part of sugar gets metabolized by every cell in your body—it's what fuels your energy. The fructose part of sugar, however, gets metabolized in your liver. If you eat a lot of sucrose from sugary foods, you're making your liver work harder because you're giving it a lot of fructose to metabolize. And if those sugary foods are sweetened with high-fructose corn syrup, your liver works even harder.

What does your liver do with all that fructose? Well, if you're already taking in plenty of calories and don't need the extra energy, your liver converts the fructose to fat. A lot of that fat ends up being stored on the spot, right there in your liver. Research tells us that a fatty liver is almost certain to cause insulin resistance and metabolic syndrome, the first steps on the road to type 2 diabetes.

You read all the scary words there: stored fat, diabetes, a vicious cycle of crashes and energy spikes. If you think that sounds like an untenable situation, it is. Sugar addicts are going to pay a price sooner or later.

Refined Carbs = Sugar

Maybe you don't eat a lot of sugary foods. In fact, maybe you don't even really *like* sweet foods. When you feel the need for a comfort food, maybe you turn to crackers, chips, and other starchy choices. And maybe when you can't get those foods, you feel anxious, irritable, and driven to find them, no matter what.

Hmmm. Sound familiar? It should. It's sugar again. Refined carbohydrates such as white flour and white rice also are converted to glucose in your bloodstream almost as soon as they're ingested. A person can become addicted to white bread, white rice, and white pasta as easily as white sugar. Being a carb addict is precisely the same as being a sugar addict.

Of course, not everyone gets addicted to sugar, just as not everyone who uses an addictive drug gets hooked on it. Some of us are simply more vulnerable to chemical dependency—on alcohol, on sugar, on drugs, on nicotine. Evidence suggests there a strong genetic tendency to addiction. Sometimes a client comes to me for help with a sugar addiction and we discover that the addiction issue lies elsewhere.

Does that mean you're an alcoholic if you're a sugar addict? Only you can say for sure. And most sugar addicts find they can kick the habit without turning to some other addictive substance as a substitute. It's not easy, and you may not succeed at first, but I know—and many other determined people know—that it can be done.

Get Ready, Get Informed

One of the best ways to prepare for cutting back on sugar calories across your diet is just to be aware of where this stuff is lurking. Read food labels carefully, looking for the words *sugar, sucrose,* and *high-fructose corn syrup* near the start of the list. To eliminate added sugars from your diet, you need to be a bit of a detective. Food manufacturers employ a lot of aliases. Sugar by any other name is just as sweet—and just as high in calories. Here are some of the words that manufacturers use on labels to hide the sugar in processed foods:

Brown sugar	Corn sugar
Corn syrup	Dextrose
Evaporated cane juice	Fructose
Fruit juice concentrate	Glucose
Golden syrup	High-fructose corn syrup (HFCS)
Honey	Lactos
Maltose	Maple syrup
Molasses	Sucrose (table sugar)
Turbinado sugar	

Copy this list onto a piece of paper and carry it with you along with the shopping list when you go to the grocery store. Use it to check out the ingredients on the food label and find those hidden sugars. If the food contains ingredients that end in -ose (sucrose), avoid it. This suffix means sugar in one form or another (Maltose, for instance, is just another name for malt sugar). There's trickery afoot. If any of the terms above is listed as one of the first five listed ingredients on the label, the food is probably high in calories and low in nutrition.

While you're avoiding added sugar, you might be tempted to try a sugar-free or reduced-sugar version of your favorite sweet foods. That's probably not a good idea. The low-sugar/no-sugar versions can carry heavy calorie loads as well. Similarly, low-fat foods often contain even more sugar than the full-fat version to make up for the lack of flavor.

Even sweeteners with low calorie loads, like aspartame, aren't without controversy. There's still a great deal we don't know about these chemicals' interactions in the human system, and there have been reports that should give you pause. In 2011, for instance, a scientific study received widespread media attention because it indicated that overreliance on diet sodas might undo many a weight-loss regimen. The study, which was presented at the American Diabetes Association Scientific Sessions, showed a direct correlation between the ingestion of diet sodas and waistline measurement in humans and blood sugar elevation in mice. No one yet has the authoritative explanation for these findings, but they underscore a basic point: you sure don't *need* to be drinking diet sodas to lose weight, and they just might hurt you.

The traps are everywhere!

But there are always ways around the traps. Diet soda drinkers can get all the fizzle and refreshment they want—from sparkling water. Crack open a Perrier instead.

How about Natural Sweeteners?

Sugar alcohols, most notably xylitol (but including any sweetener that carries the "ol" suffix), are growing in popularity since they occur in nature (even in the fibrous tissues of fruits and vegetables), have low calorie loads, are not toxic (in complex forms), and don't cause tooth decay. They generally don't raise many red flags, and by now they are found in gums, candies, chocolate, and ice cream products. As a means to combat cravings without continuing your sugar addiction, they might be helpful. Still, be careful; excessive amounts of these sweeteners can lead to plenty of gut-level complaints, including gas, diarrhea, and bloating.

Dos and Don'ts of Preparing for Detox

I know from my own experience that breaking your sugar addiction can be one of the greatest challenges you'll ever encounter. You may not succeed the first time—or the second, or the third. You will succeed in the end, however, if you detox slowly and carefully.

You don't need to give up sugar completely. In fact, a sweet food such as a favorite chocolate bar can still be on your list of must-have daily foods. What you must to do is cut back on sugar until you can be satisfied by an amount that won't damage your body or cause weight gain. Your goal is to consume sugar socially, not to feed an addiction.

It's best to begin a sugar detox quietly. Telling everyone you know about your plans is to set yourself up for failure, because you probably *will* fail, at least the first time. If the experience is embarrassing or shameful, you might decide it's easier to just stay addicted to sugar. If you announce your plans and then slip, you might resort to hiding your sugar, guiltily eating your candy bars in secret. It's no different from being a secret drinker—you're just as addicted and just as compromised by shame.

I'm very fond of the Chupa Chup, a little lollipop that delivers a small, manageable burst of sugar. It's low in calories, and it can satisfy the occasional sugar craving. But it's still a candy, and like any other sugar bomb a little indulgence should go a long way.

Yet while I was getting my nutrition degree, I was sucking on Chupa Chups like a, well, like an addict. My classmates would snicker when they saw me pop another one in my mouth. I would get defensive and say things like, "I've been in the lab for the past six hours; I need some energy." That never mollified them, because earlier in the school year I had boldly declared that sugar is addictive and bad, bad, bad, no exceptions!

Don't make announcements! At most, share your decision with someone you know will be supportive no matter what. After all, this is a very personal decision that has to come from within you.

Physical detoxification from anything addictive, cocaine or sugar, usually takes two to three weeks. It's a hard two or three weeks. People who go to clinics to detox from heroin or alcohol feel physically terrible, demand to go home, and sometimes even try to get people to smuggle them their drug. You can't sign yourself in to the clinic to detox from sugar, so the process is a bit easier (and cheaper). But because sugar is everywhere, and enjoyed by almost everyone, your challenge will still be formidable.

Take the detox process slowly, day by day. Be prepared for all those unpleasant sensations and emotions you've already experienced in the sugar cycle. Again they'll be part of the process as your brain's chemistry adjusts to lower levels of sugar intake. Also be prepared to fight with your spouse, hate your kids, and be ready to put the dog up for adoption. Stress only increases your urge to eat sugar, so think carefully about the timing of your detox. If you have a big deadline coming up at work, get through that stressful period first. If, despite your best planning, things start to go crazy while you're trying to detox, give yourself a break and wait for a better time. If you're truly motivated, you'll find a way and time, even after some false starts.

Most importantly, remember that your sugar cravings are real and won't go away just because you want them to. Instead of trying to give up sugar completely, work with your cravings while you detox.

Does detoxing that mean you'll never binge on candy, cookies, or french fries ever again? *No.* You're going to have days when you can't help yourself and simply *have* to have a lot of sugary foods. That's OK. It's not the end of the world. Remember, while eating sugar is unhealthy and being addicted to it is undesirable, you can't get arrested for driving under the influence of it. Also, remember that your ultimate goal is to be good for six days and have one day free. There are rich meals in your future (but *after* detox, during which I don't recommend taking a free day), just not so many as before!

Beginning the Sugar Detox

Sugar isn't heroin. There is no benefit to going "cold turkey" and cutting it out of your diet completely. You won't succeed in this detox by ignoring your cravings. You must work with them. This is a powerful adversary you're up against, one you probably can't banish from your life in a day. So remember: small, steady steps win this race.

The substitution method covered in chapter one should be repeated when you're ready to start cutting back sugar in earnest. For instance, if your usual breakfast is a sugary cereal, trade it in for an unsweetened whole-grain cereal topped with a spoonful of sugar. You'll still be satisfying your desire for sweet cereal first thing in the morning, but what a difference. A typical sweetened breakfast cereal has the equivalent of sixteen grams of added sugar, or four teaspoons, per serving. Cut that back to just one teaspoon on your whole-grain cereal, and you're off to a good start toward reducing your sugar intake for the day. If you usually have jam on white bread, switch to whole-grain bread and use a bit less of the jam. Try cutting back on the amount of sugar you add to your other foods as well.

And never, ever, forget to monitor your beverage intake. How much fruit juice do you usually drink in the morning? How much sweetened coffee or milk-based beverage, cappuccino lovers? And as your day rolls on, how much soda touches your lips?

If sweet beverages, especially fruit juices, are a main source of your added sugar, here's a good mantra: if you can eat it, don't drink it. Instead of the orange juice, for instance, have the orange. It normally takes *five* oranges to make one glass of juice. You'll get fewer calories, less sugar, and all the fiber that's missing from the juice. Calories saved? A medium-sized glass of orange juice has about 120 calories; a medium-sized orange has about 60 calories.

I once had a client, the president of a huge corporation, who knew he was addicted to sugary drinks but refused to give them up. This client told me he'd rather die than drink plain water. But even this hardheaded soul made progress. Gradually, he cut back by substituting diet sodas for sugary sodas and thinning his juices with just a little bit of sparkling water. I never could get him to give up his sweet drinks and juices completely; he never could make it all the way to drinking straight water. But soon he was relying on club soda with lime or lemon wedges, a far cry from the colas he was hooked on at the start. Although we didn't make it all the way to letter Z, I consider this a success story, because the client *did* cut back a great deal on sugar and lost a lot of weight.

The Next Step: Seek the Hidden Sugar

Sugar detox begins by simply not adding sugar to your already well-sugared foods. Next, you must seek out and cut back on the hidden sugars. Take time to read the small print on the packages you inspect at the market. Bring your glasses if you need them: that small print should alert you to what the contents can do to your body. A tablespoon of ketchup, for example, contains about a teaspoon of sugar, or about sixteen calories of added sugar. That doesn't sound like much, but it all adds up. A tablespoon of ketchup at lunch, another at dinner, along with the sugar that laces the prepared French dressing on your salad and the sugar that probably resides in the cream of mushroom soup, easily add gram after gram of undetected sugar to your diet. Added sugars (added by someone else, that is!) are often a primary culprit behind gradual weight gain and the frustration of uninformed dieters.

Another task is trickier, because you'll be aiming at major addiction enablers. You must cut back on food with lots of sugar and highly processed carbohydrates. Cakes, candy, ice cream, and soft drinks, all the foods you've known and loved all your life, must give up their leading roles. They can still have cameos, but if you're serious about weight loss they can no longer be a daily presence.

Some of these cutbacks can be achieved through more substitution and incremental steps. Diet soft drinks, for instance, taste sweet but have no calories. You're not eliminating your desire for a soft drink by switching to a diet option, but at least you're not getting the calorie equivalent of a liquid candy bar with each can. Instead of fake fruit juices sweetened with high-fructose corn syrup, go for real juice cut fifty-fifty with sparkling mineral water or plain, cold water.

Cut back—but, again, don't eliminate—your portions of sweet foods. To make up for the missing sweetness, substitute some fresh fruit for the rest of the portion.

Fruit is a great way to cut back on sugary foods. Imagine eating an entire box of soft, chewy chocolate cookies. All too easy, right? Now imagine eating an apple with some honey or cream. The sweetness of the apple is very satisfying, while the crunchiness gives your mouth a workout that tells your brain that you're eating real food. The fiber in the apple fills you up and also keeps the apple's natural sugar (fructose) from entering your bloodstream too quickly. You get a slow release of sugar that gives you steady energy, not highs and lows, and keeps you from feeling hungry again half an hour later. And of course, the apple is naturally full of nutrients, such as fiber and vitamin C, which you won't find in a box of cookies.

The calorie savings from cutting back on sugary foods are major. And don't underestimate the benefits of cutting down gradually. Let's say you routinely made an afternoon snack of six chocolate cookies: bad news, but nothing exceptional. Each of those chocolate cookies has about a hundred calories, about the same as a large apple. If you cut down to two cookies and add an apple, you halve this snack's calories, add some beneficial nutrients, and help your sugar detox move along. Never forget to acknowledge any accomplishment, any change in your old ways, even if it still includes a few too many sugar calories.

As your body and brain adjust to eating fewer sugary foods, keep your blood sugar on an even keel by having small, frequent snacks of high-quality carbs. Anything made with real whole grains (*not* refined white flour that's colored brown: watch out!) is helpful. So are fruits and veggies, especially if they're crunchy. If you can add a bit of protein and fat to your snack, so much the better. Good snack examples: a small handful of whole-wheat crackers with a small piece of cheese, a slice of whole-wheat toast spread with some goat cheese and a sprinkle of sunflower seeds, apple slices with some peanut butter, or low-fat plain yogurt with some fresh berries. The high-quality carbs satisfy your sugar cravings, while the protein and fat slow the release of sugar into your bloodstream and keep you from feeling hungry again too quickly.

I strongly advise investing in some healthy alternative sweeteners that give you sugar's sweet flavor without the calories. One choice is Stevia, a South American herb that's sold in the form of a powder. Gram for gram, it's much, much sweeter that table sugar, so you need to use only a tiny amount that has virtually no calories to get the same sweetness as a spoonful of sugar.

Another choice is agave nectar, made from a type of cactus that grows in Mexico (yes, tequila fans, *that* cactus). By the gram, it's actually higher in calories than table sugar, but because it's very sweet you need only a small amount to get the sweet taste.

Artificial sweeteners such as aspartame (NutraSweet) and saccharine are more widely used. They have no calories and just add sweetness to soft drinks and other foods. Use them if you must, but these are pure chemicals, and I strongly advise you aim for a diet that doesn't include them. Now, it's certainly better to drink a diet soda than one full of high-fructose corn syrup if you want to save the calories, but artificially sweetened beverages don't combat the underlying problem of sweetness addiction, because they taste just as sweet as any other beverage. Again, as an imperfect, incremental measure you can lean on these beverages as alternatives. But I wouldn't want you to get used to them.

Step by step, you need to detox from this junk. Think fast: Is it the buzz of the bubble in the soft drink that turns you on? Then try sparkling mineral water. No, don't give me attitude; just try it! You will barely notice a difference.

When Cravings Strike

Here's something to keep in mind: most sugar cravings pass in ten to fifteen minutes.

Cravings, of course, are a danger zone, an event that can undo a lot of good work quickly. I find it helps many clients (and myself) to remember that however intense a craving might be, it will be over quickly.

So how can you fight off the cravings as you detox? Get back to my country doctor's advice: move, move, move. During a brisk, twenty-minute walk, your brain will release the same endorphins that eating a candy bar will. Put physical distance between you and the temptation. It always works.

But you don't have to walk or go to the gym. *Anything* that gets you moving will help. Do some housework, dance to some music, or play with the dog. I had one client who would practice on her home pool table whenever she craved sugar. Soon she was playing a mean game of eight ball.

You have to do a little physical work to get the endorphin effect, and the effect certainly isn't as immediate as eating the chocolate is. But the activity will make you feel good—better than before the craving struck—and lower your stress level. And remember that you *only have to keep active for a brief period of time*, usually no more than a quarter of an hour. Any activity that's not eating or drinking something sweet can distract you long enough for the craving to go away. And there's another silver lining: as you cut back on sugar, you'll probably find that cravings happen less often and last for a shorter time.

Cravings can be minimized by eating a very small portion of sweet or high-carb food with every meal or snack, up until two or three hours before you go to sleep. Snacking frequently can also help to stave off a painful sugar urge. You'll gradually decrease these portions and substitute better choices until, in about a month, you find yourself eating normal, modest amounts of sugared foods without triggering strong cravings for more. In fact, many foods you used to eat in handfuls will soon taste far too sweet. You'll be ready to stop eating them after just a few bites.

So if you must calm down a sugar craving with food, do it with the smallest possible portion. Have half a chocolate bar, a small scoop of ice cream, only a couple of cookies—eat just enough to satisfy the craving without going off on a binge. This isn't a recommendation so much as advice for the bad days. If you know that even a small amount of a sugary food you love is enough to set you off, it's probably best to stay away until your palate has had time to adjust to and appreciate smaller portions. Exercise instead.

I recognize you can't always cope with a sugar craving by exercising or doing something else. In those situations (such as when you're stuck at your desk at work), try doing something with your mouth. So much of our sugar desire is really an oral fixation, a strong need to chew that originates in infancy. Chewing sugarless gum or sucking on a sugarless candy can satisfy the need without adding calories. Strongly flavored candies, especially powerful mints, seem best able to control the craving.

You can also try brushing your teeth and rinsing with a strong mouthwash; this is an unmistakable signal that grazing time is over. A little mouth cleanup is my favorite remedy when a client calls me at two in the morning in thrall to strong sugar cravings.

The Detox Reward

Your reward for going through the sugar detox is two-pronged: weight loss and better health. If you have blood sugar problems or diabetes, you already know the benefits of cutting way back on the sweet stuff. What you might not know is that cutting sugar can also help lower your cholesterol and prevent heart problems. Studies show that the people who eat the most sugar also have the lowest levels of HDL, or good cholesterol, and the highest levels of triglycerides, tiny fat droplets in the blood. Both are major risk factors for heart disease. Cut the added sugars, and you may well raise your HDL and lower your triglycerides.

There's another, delicious reward in store. Once your taste buds stop being numbed by an endless assault of sugar, you'll rediscover the true flavor of your food. (Many ex-smokers say the same thing.) When you can really enjoy the different tastes of a meal, you tend to slow down and savor your food more. When you tuck in to sweet desserts, you'll realize that after the first few bites all you can taste is the sugar. That makes it a lot easier to push the rest of the serving aside or share a dessert with someone (and win points for your generosity).

Once you've gotten over your sugar addiction, while eating sweet foods or refined carbohydrates, you may feel the impact on your blood sugar more intensely. A couple of years ago, I visited friends in Milan. Our plan was to go out for lunch and follow up with an afternoon of shopping. Because this was a special occasion, I decided to make it my free meal for the week and enjoy focaccia, which is basically a slab of thick freshly baked bread topped with herbs and thick, tasty olive oil. It was so delicious I had three big slices and felt great for about half an hour—and then, suddenly, overwhelmingly, came the carbohydrate overload, also known as carbo-coma! My friends went shopping while I staggered back to their apartment, turned on the TV, and slumped down on the couch. That's where they found me, snoring away, three hours later!

Junk Food Addiction

Of course, sugar isn't the only food addiction. Junk food—including fast foods that deliver fats and protein in addition to sugar—can be just as addicting. Our brains love foods that are high in fat, salt, and/or sugar. That's why a meal at a fast-food restaurant is so hard to resist: the classic burger, fries, and milkshake is scientifically designed to be appeal directly to our basic taste desires. Recent research conducted on rats demonstrated that consuming large amounts of junk food triggered the same brain changes as taking heroin. The "reward" circuits in the brains of obese rats (they got the junk food) were stimulated in the same manner as heroin-addicted rats. The subject that ate unlimited amounts of high-calorie, high-fat foods quickly became compulsive overeaters—they continued to chow down even after they learned that they'd receive an electric shock if they didn't stop eating. Even more striking, when the overeating rats were put back on a normal, rat-healthy diet, they went on strike and refused to eat! It took days for their brain chemicals such as dopamine to return to normal. (Sorry to cite such a cruel test of animals, but it wasn't my research!)

As with sugar addiction, detoxing from junk food is hard. Actually, in some ways, it's even harder than sugar, because highly sophisticated marketing for junk food and fast food surround us. You don't have to do any shopping at all. Just drive around any populated area, and all the restaurants, with their unforgettable logos, will pop up in your field of view. Those logos are teasers, tempters, and they work.

The method for detoxing from junk follows the same steps as sugar: Get alert to how widespread these foods are and in how many places they masquerade as "healthy" choices. Reduce your portions, and find healthier substitute foods that are convenient and enjoyable for you.

I advise you to make a real effort to avoid fast-food restaurants whenever possible. Setting foot inside one of these means your willpower must do battle with french fries, a battle you are very likely to lose. These restaurants are designed to sell you their signature foods, be it burgers or fried chicken, in large portions, and they don't offer much in the way of good alternatives. There's usually a token salad option that seems healthier. Look carefully, however, and you'll see that a salad with some toppings and dressing could actually have more calories than the burger and fries. If you must eat fast food, the salad is still the better choice for helping your junk-food addiction. It's a good way to break from the seductive taste of fatty, fried foods. It also requires some chewing, which means you take longer to eat it and feel full for longer afterward.

Sugar Success

I've helped many clients break their sugar addiction. This is a war I know you can win.

There are many success stories that I can share, but one in particular really stands out. Stella was born in Malta and ended up in Australia. Throughout her life she had fought a losing battle with sugar. She came to me overweight and diabetic.

It took eighteen months, but Stella was able to conquer her sugar addiction. I was never so proud of a patient as when she told me how her thinking had changed. "I feel great now!" she exclaimed. "I know now I can have a bite of something sweet and leave it. I don't have to eat the whole thing anymore."

That's quite an accomplishment for someone who started her detox at the age of seventy-two after decades of addiction. But Stella found the inner strength to detox from sugar. You can, too.

Summary

- *Addiction to sugar and simple carbohydrates is commonplace, and is a leading cause of obesity and a host of health problems.*

- *Be a sugar detective—read food labels to discover the hidden sugar in common food items, and watch your weight melt away.*

- *Begin detox from sugar by eating smaller portions of sugary and high-carb foods at every meal. Eliminating sugar cold turkey is a shock to the system and may backfire.*

- *Detox from sugar and simple carbs slowly, gradually replacing sugary and high-carb foods with food of better nutritional quality and food you really like.*

- *Cope with sugar cravings by becoming involved in a physical activity or by using tricks to distract yourself.*

Chapter Three

THE THREE DIET
PERSONALITIES

There's more than one person up in our heads. Depending on the situation, one or the other personality might come to the foreground. In my two decades of work, I've concluded there's a strong correlation between the personality that falls in love and the one that manages our relationship with food.

It's no surprise to me. Changing your relationship with food is a lot like breaking up with a lover. Of course, this won't be a breakup, per se; you'll simply be choosing a new, healthier approach, one that acknowledges your natural love of food, even the so-called "bad" foods, and doesn't attempt to shut them out of your life.

As it so often goes between lovers, the big issue here is about control. To have a healthy bond with a partner, we need to feel some degree of control, at least most of the time. Trouble often starts when one person has too much, the other not enough. These imbalanced situations can go on for years; they can deepen to the point where leaving is the only route back to happiness. My program is designed for you regain some happiness.

I've come to identify three basic personality types when it comes to food: Decision Makers, Advice Seekers and Victims. Sometimes, a client is cut-and-dried, what-you-see-is-what-you-get; they're completely one personality type without even a hint of influence from the others. Other clients have a dominant personality type that is influenced, occasionally, by one of the others, or both. These are general guidelines, but I find it very helpful for my clients to be aware, early on, of their psychological makeup.

So what personality type are you? Here's a quick introduction.

The Decision Maker

Decision Makers aren't too interested in the backstory. They spend little time on the causes of a problem. They focus on solutions. They detect the problem (and if it's extra weight, the detection process is pretty much immediate), find the solution, and apply it. This is the person who might run from A to Z in record time with barely a hurdle to cross. Right after this person has made a decision to make a change, she is well on her way to making it.

You probably know from experience that when your Decision Maker friend asks you to lunch to discuss her boyfriend problem, that boyfriend is probably halfway out the door already (because she pushed him there!). By the end of the lunch she'll have concluded that the romance is unhealthy and formulated a plan for packing up that weekend. And she'll do it. If she sets a deadline, she'll stick to it. And the next time you see her, probably she'll be full of stories about the move, her latest flirtations, and expectations for the future. The message is clear: the boyfriend is gone and not even missed.

This personality type has no trouble making the commitment to weight loss. Once she's got the idea, she's ready to go through the process, no matter what.

36

One of my favorites was Jasmine. She came in one day, sat down, and announced, "Diana, I've heard about you. I know you want commitment from your clients. I did some research on you, and let me tell you—you got the job! I want, I mean, I *need* to lose ten kilos. I did my research on that, too. So I need you to tell me how to lose weight, and keep it off. Give me a course about how my body works. Whatever you say, I will do it."

I don't think I ever had an easier client! She didn't just listen, either; she'd come prepared with lots of good, informed questions, and when satisfied with the explanations she would go off and do what she was told.

Amazing!

She lost her weight, and she has kept it off.

When a Decision Maker is in high gear, she might not need to do any more than read this book. She'll zero in on Z and plow through any obstacles in record time. Sugar detox? Check. Exercise? She took a gym membership before she started the program and cleared three hours of her working week to make sure she goes. The Decision Maker, you see, has her physical energy and willpower yoked together. Her belief is so strong it gets her through most rough patches before she's even noticed they exist!

Decision Makers aren't infallible, of course. Because they tend to be impulsive, they sometimes are vulnerable to bad marketing and fads. Their enthusiasm is great, but they also can run quite a ways down the wrong road before they notice they're lost. I've met Decision Makers who were so confused after years of taking diet pills, eating every other day, and other extreme weight-loss measures that it was necessary for them to stop and reflect before they embraced my methods. Like everyone else, the Decision Makers need the support of informed professionals and reliable information to effect change on their eating habits.

So if you're a go-getter, keep reading! I know you were ready to get started on your weight-loss program yesterday, but make sure you have a well-thought-out plan before you begin.

Some people embody the Decision Maker in every area of their lives; others always seem to sneak out of making any firm commitments. But I believe we all have this can-do spirit inside of us, and it probably has sparked every one of my successful clients, no matter how I first sized them up.

The Advice Asker (and Follower)

Generally, this is the friend who invites you out, tells you all about the problems she's having in her romance, and asks what you think. "Should I leave him/her or should I stay? Jade says I should leave, but then Francesca tells me I should stay. I'm so confused. What should I do?"

So you give your earnest opinion. She listens gravely. Later, you discover that the very next day, she asked *another* friend whether it was time for her to leave.

When it comes to food and weight loss, the Advice Asker has heard every opinion and read every study (and shred of gossip) about the right way to diet. The essential difference between this approach and that of the Decision Maker perhaps isn't what you think. It's not that the Advice Asker doesn't ask questions: she *always* has questions. But she doesn't follow through and critically evaluate all the information she receives. The "best diet" usually is the one highlighted in the current issue of a fashion magazine. "This is how Lindsay Lohan lost her weight!" "It's all about the 'Apple Diet'! Just eat three apples a day, and nothing else, for a month!" Advice Askers get plenty of information, all right, but they don't often stop to sift through it. And they never really commit to a firm choice.

Although many diet out of habit, Advice Askers tend to move on to the next New Thing when the going gets tough, because they're convinced there's a quick fix out there. While it's true that fads always manage to pull in some Decision Makers, they usually pull in *lots* of Advice Askers, who are always ready to jump on a passing bandwagon.

I've learned that you really can't have any affect on these personality types by offering yet more advice; you're just joining the crowd. When they come to me as clients, I make sure that the details of my program are clearly described and understood. Then, I simply tell them, "Do what your heart tells you."

Every body is unique, and the ultimate authority on its function and peculiarities is the person living inside of it. Advice Askers simply have taken a sensible approach to an extreme. As Decision Makers know, sound advice is necessary. But my program is about ownership: of your weaknesses, your strengths, and your happiness. Advice Askers who embrace it must first embrace their own authority.

The Victim

In romance, the Victim doesn't need advice about staying or going. She's been wronged. She knows she needs to go. But she's also made up her mind that she can't.

This personality is ingenious at finding justifications for inaction and excuses for why nothing in her life has changed. Yet she's always ready to leave; she's going to leave *this time*. Just like every other time in the last five years (or ten or twenty).

Still, at the lunch when she makes her announcement, you strike a positive tone. "Great," you say. "Go for it, even if you're scared. After all, you've known this is what you need to do for years."

That, of course, is the step too far. She gives you a sharp look. "It's not so easy, you know." And then comes the list. The ironclad, unassailable list of reasons why she can't do what she says she needs to do! He needs her. She can't survive on her own. She's too old to find someone else. They were made for each other.

Victims long ago figured out why they can never achieve the healthy body they want. They are quite aware that their lives desperately require some change, and they often are frightened by the health risks of remaining over-weight. But just as in love, there's always a reason why they can't lose weight, a reason that leaves them blameless.

The Victim's relationship with food often is as toxic as her romantic engagements. Her methods are very different, but like the Advice Seeker she takes no responsibility for her plight, and so she is stuck with it.

When a Victim first sits down with me, often the explanation of her condition can last an hour or more. Her metabolism is slow (usually, she doesn't know what "metabolism" really is, but she knows it's slow!). Her body is resistant to weight loss. She tries harder than her "skinny bitch" friend, who can always lose weight if she wants. She's doesn't have the money for a successful effort. Her mother is too bossy/controlling/depressed/demanding, and always sabotages her. Work is too stressful. Every time she tries to change her lifestyle, a family member, friend, or colleague makes fun.

Remember that we all have our blind spots: victims often have blacked out enormous chunks of their personality and circumstances. Many of them deal with their work lives and other responsibilities just fine. But when it comes to food and weight, they believe the odds are all stacked against them. Other people are lucky, and they aren't.

The Victim is just as susceptible to bad marketing as the Decision Maker and Advice Asker, but that's the least of her problems. Of far greater concern is that she has ingeniously sabotaged every effort to change her relationship with food before it even began.

In the initial stages of working with Victims, I often feel more like a psychologist than an expert in nutrition and health. But the start is exactly the moment when fad diets fail. People who refuse to combat their blind spots, who remain passive participants in their lives, will never sustain a healthy weight. Only a Decision Maker can get all the way from A to Z.

But don't feel shame, Victims! Shame is just another means to keep your blind spots in operation. Today, I *know* you can really start thinking about what you eat, how you feel about it, and how you can take control of it. There's a Decision Maker inside you waiting to get out. After twenty years of working with Victim personalities, I'm confident we can snap you out of your old cycle.

Taking Control

Maybe you think I have a preference for the Decision Maker personality, but that's only true insofar as it's much easier for me to work with them! Look at it this way: Decision Makers usually are starting the A-to-Z process a little further along than Advice Askers and Victims. They skip a few intro letters because, true to their name, *they already have decided that they can succeed.* It's the one given that the other two personality types don't allow for; each, in its way, assumes the worst—failure—and pretty much guarantees that result.

This is one reason why I will so often remind you that yes, you can do something. Once you believe that you're capable, you can keep going. Since you're human, there's no guarantee that you won't have setbacks and complications, but that belief in yourself will provide energy when it's time to get back up and start again.

We're all unique. But deciding that yes, we're capable of weight loss and controlling the food relationship is the first and most important step for every one of us.

Rebecca is a successful business manager, a self-made woman, proud of her career achievements. At work she is respected as a colleague and a boss. She's been overweight for about ten years.

Which Personality Type is Rebecca?

Since her career took off, Rebecca has been frustrated by the ineffectiveness of her dieting attempts. When she travels, she takes along magazines and books that champion one weight-loss method or another. She's envious of her slender friends and frequently asks them what they're doing to keep their weight in balance.

When pressed, Rebecca will say it's impossible for her to plan a moderate diet because she's working so much and relying on hotel and airplane food. She doesn't have time to figure out the best way to eat. When she's home, she's too tired to go shopping. Plus, she has the money to eat out or order takeout most nights, so she does. She never learned how to cook. All her skinny friends cook, she says.

A: At work, Rebecca is a Decision-Maker all the way. But when it comes to her weight, she loses that alluring confidence. She's a little too anxious to rely on the advice of others, and when push comes to shove she actually goes the Victim route! Rebecca is blinding herself to the fact that she can approach her life with food as she approaches work. Once she does, she'll be a great candidate for raising her weight-loss IQ in rapid fashion.

Summary

- *There are three diet personalities—the Decision Maker, the Advice Asker, and the Victim—and it's important to understand which one you are. Knowing which diet personality you are will help you to eliminate blinds spots and move on.*

Chapter Four

ARE YOU OVERWEIGHT?

Are you overweight? And if you are, how overweight are you?

Simple questions, right? Not so fast. With all the information coming our way it doesn't take long to lose sight of a reliable definition of what your healthy weight is. Mirrors judge us, cameras lie, doctors get too casual with the "fit fat" description, the girl next door always looks slimmer, and what's in the number that comes up on the scale, anyway?

As it turns out, determining a healthy weight may be more like judging beauty than we think. There's always a subjective element to the calculation.

Think back to the personality types we discussed in the last chapter. Naturally your personality has a role in determining if you're overweight and, if the answer is yes, by how much.

The Decision Maker probably is going to stick to the basics. She doesn't feel as light on her feet as she'd like. Her clothes don't fit, or she has a hard time finding clothes she likes. Hard numbers will drive her to seek help; she'll unearth some definition of what her "ideal" weight is for her height, and if she's over it, she'll take steps.

The Advice Asker will need to ask a dozen people if her ass is fat. When they politely say no, she'll persist: "Are you sure?" She'll keep this up until someone is honest (or fed up) enough to tell her she is fat. Then it will be on to advice about what diet to follow. On she'll go, becoming a bit more confused and uncertain about how overweight she really is. Sooner or later, she'll go back to what she knows: asking for advice!

The Victim *knows* that she's overweight and will obsess over her need to slim down. Action, real action, of course, will be out of the question.

In truth, many people believe they are horribly overweight when in fact they're only about eleven pounds/five kilograms too heavy, which really isn't very much. Some believe their ideal weight is much lower than it should ever be, opening them up to the threat of eating disorders.

If you don't know what a healthy weight range is for you, you won't know how much to lose to get there. So it's important that you have a few means of evaluating where you are; used together, these measurements will give you a pretty accurate read on your weight and how far from a healthy weight it is or isn't. There are three calculations and then a tried-and-true method you might have forgotten about.

Using the Body Mass Index (BMI)

The standard medical approach is to calculate your body mass index, or BMI, and compare it to a chart that gives weight ranges for your height; this index is meant to determine if you're normal weight, overweight, or obese. Since your BMI is based on your height and weight (and is for adults only, not teenagers or children), it's a good way to learn about the how wide your "normal weight" range is.

The formula is fairly simple:

Body Mass Index (BMI) = Weight kg / Height m²

In metric units, it's your weight divided by the square of your height. Take your weight in kilograms and divide it by your height in meters, times your height in meters (in other words, your height in meters squared). In US or imperial measurements, multiply 703 by your weight in pounds and divide it by your height in inches times your height in inches (your height in inches squared). The resulting figure is your BMI.

If you don't like to do your own math, you can calculate your BMI online in US or metric measurements (www.nhlbisupport.com/bmi/). For US measurements, you can also just look for your BMI in the US BMI chart (pdf: www.nhlbi.nih.gov/guidelines/obesity/bmi_tbl.pdf.) These sites will tell you where your number falls in the weight range for your height.

Charts won't mean much, however, if you don't learn more about those weight ranges, so let's mock up a hypothetical case—"Sarah"—and run her numbers.

Let's say that Sarah is 5'7"/1.75 centimeters tall and weighs 215 pounds/98 kilograms.

A. Multiply her height times her height. This is 1.75 x 1.75.

This equals 3.06.

B. We're going to divide Sarah's weight, 98 kilograms, by 3.06.

This equals 32.

So Sarah's BMI is 32. Compare that number to the range below. According to the chart, she's technically obese, on the low end of that chart segment. Find out your number and see where you fall:

Under 18.5:	**Underweight**
18.5 to 24.9:	**Normal weight**
25 to 29.9:	**Overweight**
30 to 39.9:	**Obese**
40 and up:	**Morbidly obese (more than fifty kilograms over your ideal body weight)**

OK, now it's important to consider just how *wide* these BMI ranges are in real life. For example, a woman who is five feet five inches tall has a normal weight range—a BMI of 18.5–24.9—between 114 and 144 pounds, a thirty-pound range! This tells you two things: the definition of a "healthy" weight might not be as narrow as you think, and the BMI does have a few limitations.

If you are 5'5", you probably feel it's desirable to be closer to 114 pounds than 144. But, depending on other factors, you might still be at a healthy weight if you're close to the higher number.

This is important to keep in mind when you set your weight-loss goals. Sure, you might think the lower end of the range is an ideal target, but if you aim for a higher number, you will, of course, reach your goal a lot faster. (And then you can always revise your goals!) Remember, the ultimate *Yes, You Can* goal is to have a happy, healthy weight that is sustainable. You're aiming to feel better and look better.

For some people, a happy weight isn't within the normal weight range of the BMI chart. I can still work productively with these clients; many scientific studies have shown that if you're overweight, losing just 10 percent of your body weight is enough to positively impact your health. That modest loss's effect on your looks also can be considerable.

Beyond these personal preferences, the BMI measurement has other limitations. It doesn't take into account

* your sex,
* your age,
* your build,
* your health,
* how muscular you might be.

People who have lost weight because of illness, for example, may be at the lower end of the "healthy weight" category and need to put back on a few pounds. Then, there's my friend Daniel, a bodybuilder who has well-developed muscles and minimal body fat. His height is 1.72 centimeters (about 5'6½") and he weighs 194 pounds/88 kilograms. Plug those numbers into a BMI index and Daniel is obese! Obviously, he's anything but.

A doctor, over-relying on BMI, might tell you your weight is on the high end of the "normal" spectrum. But if you're wheezing when you walk up a few stairs, you've probably fallen through a BMI loophole (as I believe many people in the "fit fat" category do). Or perhaps you were at the middle of the normal BMI range five years ago, but now you're at the high end. That's a situation you probably will want to deal with.

Using the Waist-Hip Ratio (WHR)

WHR is a simpler computation, and all you need to figure it is a tape measure. It can help determine the severity of the health risks your extra pounds might carry. Research has shown that waist measurements of more than thirty-five inches for women and above forty for men substantially increase the risk of heart disease, diabetes, high blood pressure, and some types of cancer (such as colon, breast, and prostate).

You'll take two measurements; first run the tape around your waist at its smallest point—around your torso and just above your belly button. Then, measure your hips at their widest point, which will be the widest part of your buttocks. Divide your waist measurement (the smaller number) by your hip measurement (the larger number). The number you come up with is your WHR.

Let's say your waist is thirty-five inches and your hips are forty-six inches. That gives you a WHR of 0.76. A WHR of less than one means you're a pear shape: if you have excess weight, you're carrying it in your thighs and buttocks. A WHR higher than one means you're an apple shape: You're carrying your extra weight in your belly area.

So is it better to be a pear or an apple? There's some evidence that pear-shaped people are less likely to encounter the health problems that come with being overweight or obese, but the research jury is still out on this one. In other words, a low WHR isn't ironclad insurance against health problems.

Here's what the WHR tells you, generally, about your health risks:

Male	Female	Health Risk Based on WHR
0.95 or below	0.80 or below	Low risk/Normal weight
0.96 to 1.0	0.81 to 0.85	Moderate risk /Normal weight—Overweight
1.0+	0.85+	High risk/Overweight

Using the Body Fat Percentage (BFP)

BFP is an extremely complicated calculation, so you'll certainly want to use an online calculator unless you really love running numbers. Breaking down the calculation is beyond this book's scope, so instead I'll point you toward an efficient aid at www.everydayhealth.com/toolkit/body-fat-calculator.aspx.

This measurement will tell you how much body fat you have and compare it to your lean muscle mass. Optimal BFP varies depending on your age and sex.

You must have an accurate read on your height and weight to begin. Then, using a tape measure, find the circumference of your neck, waist, and hips. Plug this data into the online calculator.

This chart gives you the healthy range of BFP ratios:

Male	Female	Age Range
8–19 percent	21–32 percent	Under age 39
11–24 percent	23–35 percent	Over age 39

Now you have three ratios that, taken together, will provide you with a fairly accurate estimate of how overweight you are and the health risks you face as a result. They aren't meant to replace your common sense and innate knowledge of how your body feels and looks; they should help you better understand your body's messages and determine the goals you will set for yourself.

Once you have the figures, write them down. You'll refer back to them often, especially once you're making real strides forward with weight loss.

But in my program, you aren't done with measurements. In fact, you'll be taking a measurement every single day.

That's right: I am an advocate of the daily weigh-in, a practice that has grown so controversial it requires some background and explanation.

Scale, Scale on the Floor

As the world's population grows heavier and heavier, standards change: what was once thought of as XL rapidly is becoming L, which will soon be M (unless a bad trend reverses). Conventional wisdom comes to be judged as foolhardy.

Listen to this:

"Your body is made of water, and the fluids in your body will fluctuate all the time, so don't weigh yourself."

"It will make you feel worse if you weigh yourself and the scale shows you are not losing weight but actually putting some on."

"You should just weigh yourself once a week and not get obsessed with the scale."

Do these statements sound familiar? In the seventies and eighties, jumping on the bathroom scale in the morning after a nice poop, a shower, and brushed teeth was not considered an obsession; it was the norm. And it made sense.

Today, the majority of weight-loss consultants tell their clients to weigh in once a week. I believe this is a due to confusion over the purpose of the daily weigh-in. Years of fads, misinformation, and bad advice have pulled our consciousness away from common sense.

The fact is, the scale is like a tough-talking but loyal friend. It doesn't always tell you what you want to hear, but it gives you the truth, *so long as you check in with it regularly!*

Scales don't lie (as long as they're functioning properly; I advise you to invest in a brand-new digital model before you begin this program). But, like computers, they can't think: it's up to you to do the thinking and to put the numbers into context. One individual weigh-in doesn't tell you much, and it's true that on any given day there may be temporary factors contributing to a sudden weight spike. But people who use the scale daily aren't interested in *one* number. They're putting together a *sequence* of numbers that is accurate, informative, and almost always in sync with how they feel.

Let's say you weigh 154 pounds/70 kilograms on Monday and wait until the following Sunday to weigh in again. Now, the scale says 158.5 pounds/72 kilograms. What does this number mean? It could mean a lot of things—some normal, some not—but you have no way of isolating a cause because you simply don't have enough information. You don't know what your body was doing the rest of the week.

People who weigh in once a week or never at all are too detached from their bodies. They're keeping themselves in the dark about its routine functions, so there's less opportunity to know for sure if there's a problem. The daily weigh-in provides the information you need. And it keeps you accountable.

In the seventies and eighties, when obesity was not yet at epidemic levels, the scale helped many women keep slim, especially in Europe; they weighed themselves each day. When they saw that the number was consistently going up, they ate less and healthier and exercised more. Along with calorie counting (more on that in a minute), the weigh-in helped people understand what they were putting into their body each day, and how much. There were no complicated calculations involved. Armed with some basic personal information and knowledge of food and calories amounts, many enjoyed the benefits of this system. And for a long time, it *really* worked.

Ask any bodybuilder if he or she uses the scale. Of course! Bodybuilders aren't concerned with how well their jeans fit or if they look bigger; those are unreliable indicators. So they weigh themselves to maintain awareness of their progress and their bodies' natural functions.

Weight is like your body's water content; it fluctuates. Can you determine how much it fluctuates if you're on the scale just once a week? If the number is high, that day is ruined. But it's entirely possible this is a temporary spike caused by fluid retention. It happens to everyone, but without other recent numbers for comparison, how can you know what's really going on?

The weight of the average person can fluctuate as much as seven pounds/three kilograms, up and down, on a regular basis. That's a lot of weight! And it has nothing to do with adding fat. It's just the body doing what it always does.

The primary culprit behind many of these fluctuations—bodily fluids—is sensitive to the volume of fiber in your diet, salt retention, hormonal shifts (particularly during the menstrual cycle), and byproducts of the digestive process, namely pee, poo, and gas. A salty meal in the evening could cause fluid retention that bumps your weight a kilo by the next morning. Now, if you were so unlucky as to make that morning the only one in ten when you stepped on the scale, what will you think? Suddenly, a dinner at which you might have been very careful about what you ate and drank looks like a diet-buster.

Women can gain up to 5 pounds/2.2 kilograms in retained water during the week before their periods. Many become constipated at this time, too, which adds on a kilo or more of poo. Again, if you are sporadic about your weigh-ins, a normal monthly buildup of bloat and poo, *not* fat, can look awfully like bad weight gain, even when you're conscientious about your diet!

How many despondent women have fallen back into unrestricted consumption of fried chicken and ice cream because they made this type of mistake? More than I care to count.

You need to see these weight fluctuations for yourself. If you take the time to understand your body's pattern of weight fluctuation, slow weight loss, plateaus, and even small gains won't leave you discouraged. And, in the event that you truly *have* gained unwanted weight, you'll have solid proof.

And that's the tough love in action. The scale does impart bad news when your weight-loss routines get shaky. I see this as yet another reason to get used to those daily consultations. Hiding from your weight gain is a lot like leaving your banking and credit card statements unopened when you know your finances are in disarray. Here's one way out: open your bills and deal with them. When you weigh in daily, you own your weight-loss success, or the lack of it.

Once you have a daily routine in place, your unique weight-fluctuation pattern will quickly reveal itself to you. You'll be informed and accountable. When you've had a stressful week and reverted to your old, sugar-centric eating habits, the scale will tell you. And you'll have the information you need to get back on track.

To really drive home the value of a scale, I'll tell a tale on myself. Many years ago, when I, too, had no idea of how useful scales are and never stood on one, I gained thirty-one pounds/fourteen kilograms—and never noticed! After all, my jeans still fit. No one noticed, not me, not my family, not my boyfriend, and certainly not my jeans! This exemplifies why you can't get by without the scale's daily report. Numbers aren't glamorous, but they hold up much better than our subjective observations ever do.

Here's one reason you can't gauge weight by how well your pants fit: clothing stretches, especially clothes made out of newer synthetics that are designed to have some give. Know, too, that you can't make conclusions if the size you fit into has changed. Sizes vary widely depending on the manufacturer or designer; what's a large in one brand might be a small in the next. Sizes keep shrinking, too. I used to be a small-medium, but today I'm an extra-extra small, yet my weight has remained constant! Forget about your clothes, and get that scale.

Find Your Weight Common Denominator

So how long does it take to discover what your average weight is?

If you get on the scale every morning, two weeks is enough time to determine your weight common denominator. This simply is the number the scale reports most often in that two-week period. If you are 154 pounds/70 kilograms on Monday morning, you'll likely see fluctuations over the next fourteen days, but if 154 pounds/70 kilograms is the number you most often see in the morning, that is your weight common denominator.

In my program, a 154-pound person might dip down to 149.5 and swing up as far as 159. If that person has absorbed my message, she won't be alarmed by the 159 report; she'll know this is just part of the regular cycle. But if, in the next two weeks, 149.5 has become the new weight common denominator, she'll know she's making good progress.

Of course, the longer your weigh-in log becomes, the impressive, steady progress will appear. I advise that you make the morning weigh-in as automatic as brushing your teeth, but even if you only commit to two months with the scale you will know a great deal more about how your body functions. The aberrations will stand out as narrow spikes on a chart, and a weight denominator shift, from say 180 pounds/82 kilograms to 169/77 will stand out clearly as a downward path in the right direction.

And when you see an upward spike, remember that there are several likely culprits:

1.   Constipation. Poo retains fluids and has weight! It's also one of the reasons you could find it difficult to lose weight.
2.   You had a salty dinner and are bloated with retained water.
3.   If you're a woman, you're close to your period or have your period.
4.   You're using someone else's scale, and it's not as accurate as yours!

Your Metabolism Is Part of the Numbers Game, Too

Diet books and diet plans often talk about your "metabolism" without ever explaining exactly what it is. Worse yet, for many people, metabolism is a fuzzy concept that explains how their "slender" friends magically put away any and all forbidden foods without ever gaining weight: "Look at her! She can eat whatever she wants and never gain a pound!" I could scream every time I hear these comments, except that I'd have screamed myself hoarse a long time ago!

Understanding generally what your metabolism is and what affects it is key to understanding how to lose your weight and what challenges you might be facing.

A body's metabolism is a set of chemical reactions that convert fuel—what we eat and drink—into the energy that's needed to keep the body and mind active. There are a number of factors that contribute to or detract from its efficiency, including age, gender, and genetics. But what you eat—which is entirely up to you—is a huge factor. Your metabolism may be a series of chemical functions, but you're a living person, not a chemistry lab. Pay attention to the external factors first!

The idea that all those skinny people are "just lucky" is nonsense. You may be convinced that the metabolic gods favor them because, in your experience, they aren't careful about what they eat, and maybe they enjoy foods you know to be bad news. But you aren't with those people all day. Some of them have jobs—as personal assistants, servers, or trainers—that burn more calories than the demands of your desk job. Some buy high-calorie foods but eat them sparingly, or never finish what they buy. Some of them (hold your breath) are younger than you. There could be many more explanations, but luck isn't one of them.

Once you have learned the details of my program, you'll guess that the skinny girl eating a doughnut at work isn't living on doughnuts alone. Probably, she's feeding her metabolism many more "clean foods"[1] when you're not around.

Unfortunately, you can't underestimate the role age plays in the metabolic equation. Your metabolism was high when you were a child and a teenager, but once you hit adulthood it almost certainly began to slow down. With the

---

1. "Clean food" is an expression I use very often. It means food that is not elaborately prepared or heavily processed. This can be something like grilled chicken breasts with salad and a sweet potato, or salmon and vegetables with a sprinkle of cheese on the top. No frying in loads of oil and no heavy sauces. We'll talk more about these foods in Chapter Five.

slowdown comes a natural loss of muscle mass, even among people who make an effort to stay fit and toned. And the lost muscle is replaced by—guess what—body fat.

I know, not fair, is it? I wish I could say it wasn't true, but starting in her thirties, the average person loses about five pounds of muscle each decade, unless she balances the loss with the right kind of exercise and attention to diet. The fact is, the older you get, the more exercise you'll need, and you'll need to eat clean food pretty much throughout six-and-a-half days (still leaving open your free meal).

So start practicing now! Once you've made the effort to change your habits, you will find it difficult to *not* to eat clean and exercise.

Never mind your skinny, carefree (and probably young) friend. Look at Jane Fonda instead. She's in her seventies, and she looks the way she does because she has been jumping up and down, promoting fitness videos and healthy food from before I was born! Of course, she's a wealthy actress, so it's easy for people to chalk up her fine form to cosmetic surgery. Don't believe it. There are a lot of rich women in their late seventies who look *nothing* like Jane Fonda. They tend to look like strange creatures with bumpy fat left behind by cosmetic surgeons. Jane Fonda looks healthy. Her fantastic posture is the result of years of hard work, exercising, and eating well. All the cosmetic surgery in the world won't hide a lifetime of poor eating choices and lack of exercise.

Obviously, by watching what you eat and maintaining a regular exercise program, you can fight this natural aging process, up to a point. But even lean-as-a-whippet triathletes will find their body composition changing as they age. Like everyone else, their muscle mass is more metabolically active than fat and needs much more energy to sustain itself. And so, when it's replaced by fat, those triathletes burn fewer calories. Those pesky fat cells mostly just sit around, waiting to be needed (which is a throwback to our hunter/gatherer ancestors, who needed to store fat to protect against starvation in times of famine, which certainly were a lot more common before McDonald's came to Earth).

So even if your diet is unchanged, as you age you might need, perhaps, one hundred fewer calories every day without knowing it. That can add up to a weight gain of nine pounds/four kilograms in a year—a lot of weight for you, innocently eating as you always did! It's not fair, but that's what bodies do.

But you know what to do. Once that scale is in the bathroom, waiting for you, there's no excuse for getting caught unaware!

Summary

- *There are a number of methods to discover if you are truly overweight as well as understand how much weight you need to lose to achieve your ideal body.*

- *Weigh yourself at the same time every day in order to understand your present weight fluctuations and your weight common denominator; there are several factors that affect weight on a day-to-day basis.*

Chapter Five

GET SMART: RAISE YOUR NUTRITIONAL IQ

No, I'm not saying you're dumb. Not at all.

You probably show off your smarts daily, whether you recognize it or not. Many of my weight-loss clients are intelligent, well-educated people. Their high IQs serve them well professionally, but when it comes to nutrition and exercise, they often know surprisingly little. A big part of my job is raising their nutrition IQ. That's what we'll accomplish in this chapter.

A good grasp of the basics is essential for an achievable diet plan. You need to understand how your body uses food and how quickly it manages to use it. This will make you much savvier about hunger pangs (and other impulses that sneakily imitate hunger).

Don't underestimate the value of this; when you can expect real hunger to strike, you can be that much more confident cutting out those first unnecessary calories.

BTW—What's a Calorie Really?

Unbelievably, there are trends in weight loss that trivialize this question. When it comes to calories, I've heard some dieters and professionals say, "Just don't bother counting them."

What nonsense. A working definition of a calorie is essential to raising your nutrition IQ.

A calorie is the basic unit used to measure the energy value of a food. In other words, every food is a vehicle for a certain amount of energy, and it contains a certain number of calories that the body will metabolize one way or the other.

That's the shorthand description. We could spend some time getting into the chemistry of joules and energy, but what's more important to know is how much energy you need to complete your daily activities.

For example, you use about 130 calories (about the number of calories contained in a small baked potato) if you walk at an average pace for thirty minutes. Who knew a baked potato had such staying power? Many people, when they hear how much activity is required to burn off the calories they consume, think that weight loss is just about controlling calorie intake. Your BMR says you need 1,700 calories? Just take in 1,200! Cut 500 calories out and you're golden! Who needs exercise?

Nice try, couch potatoes! But the truth is, cutting your calorie intake and burning calories through exercise are *not* the same thing! Calorie cutters will soon get tired of all the deprivation, and they should. It's true that your weight gain in part was due to eating too much. But it also happened because your body's balance of consuming and burning fuel (that is, exercising) was tipped too far toward consumption. You need to burn more to achieve balance again, and we'll talk about how, and why, in chapter ten.

There are plenty of weight-loss fads I believe are useless, and some are harmful; that doesn't mean all the information they provide is bad. If you've ever used a program to try to lose weight, you've probably counted calories before. Even if you've never tried dieting, you've surely noticed all the nutritional value labeling that comes on boxes of packaged food. It's there because we're supposed to read it! Oh yes, the secret is out! And guess what? I designed my program around calorie counting, too. So, what's the difference?

There are two differences, actually. My clients learn not just how many calories foods contain, but also which foods are suitable substitutions when you can't find something on your planned menu. The whole idea here is for you to have the knowledge and the power: Don't rely overly on dietitians and nutritionists, Advice Seekers and Victims! You don't need a pro to tell you that if an apple (about one hundred calories) isn't what you want, you can switch it out for an orange, a small pear, six strawberries, and so on.

Let's imagine a day when you snatch a doughnut, a day when eating isn't free. Panicking won't help! Rather, I want you to learn how to rebalance your calorie intake for the rest of the day by eating lightly and/or exercising. But to do that, you need to know what foods can be appropriate substitutes and, ideally, where you can find them.

Sure, you can pay to have meals delivered to you from profitable weight-loss programs. You can pay to go to weight-loss meetings. But listen up, Victims on tight budgets: *You can do it all yourself.*

Are You Hungry?

One of the goals of weight loss is so simple that it bears repeating, because it gets lost under all the numbers: you must learn how to eat when you're hungry and to stop eating when you're full.

You can't find a much simpler directive than that. But hunger isn't so simple anymore. In our era of abundance, it's hard for most affluent people to know what hunger *really* is.

Hunger is the driving force behind almost everything we do. Above all else, we need to eat to stay alive. By now, however, food, hunger, and eating are more than mere survival mechanisms. Food, far more than we need, is everywhere. And we're eating for reasons that have nothing to do with actual hunger—constantly.

On top of that, today we live with incredibly sophisticated marketing for processed foods, fast foods, and restaurants. You're told that eating this food makes you feel good, so why not have some more? It's very hard to escape these messages.

Learning to Recognize Hunger

I often ask people how they know when they're hungry. Many look confused: they know hunger when they feel it. Do they feel it often? Of course, they say. Then I tell them that they probably can't distinguish true hunger from other sensations. And by the same principle, they can't recognize a feeling of fullness.

Why is this? We eat for so many (often lousy) reasons that many people simply can't recognize true hunger any more. In fact, true hunger is a rare event for people of means.

You probably eat three meals a day and have at least one snack in between, and another in the evening before bed. When was the last time you went for more than a few hours without eating something? (No, the day before your colonoscopy doesn't count.)

The clock can trigger "hunger pangs" even if our stomachs aren't empty; we're just like Pavlov's dogs hearing the food bell. I also find that the longer a person has been following and discarding diet plans, the less able he or she is to recognize hunger. Her senses have become disorientated by years of following plans and responding to those bells, instead of listening to her body.

It's no surprise that when a dieter ends yet another plan, whatever it is, he's helpless. The plan kept him on track; without it, he can't control his appetite—he's forgotten how, if he ever knew!

Hunger/Fullness

It's time for you to differentiate between hunger and other sensations, such as thirst, boredom, anxiety, or tiredness. Like so much else in the weight-loss industry, there are many metrics for rating a person's degree of hunger. I've simplified the process; I suggest that you rate your hunger on a scale of one to seven:

1. You're not hungry—you're ravenous. Hopefully that's good food on your plate, because you're going to eat it regardless.

2. You're moderately hungry—you're ready to eat a good, nutritious meal.

3. You're mildly hungry—you're *beginning* to want something to eat. Dinner's in an hour? Good, by then you'll really be looking forward to eating.

4. You're neither hungry nor full. Sure, you could eat something; you wouldn't turn down a snack. But the fact is, there's nothing wrong with waiting until the next meal.

5. You're slightly full—you just ate and you feel satisfied. A cup of coffee? Why sure, but you'll pass on dessert.

6. You're very full—you're at the end of a big meal, and you don't want to eat again for a while. Until, say, tomorrow. You really don't want *anyone* counting calories right now.

7. You're overstuffed—you ate way too much, and your stomach feels distended and uncomfortable. Bloating, cramps, bad news on the scale tomorrow: some way or another you'll pay for this.

Unlike the scale on your floor, this one is completely subjective. It's based entirely on how you feel at the moment, not on how many calories you did or didn't eat. Your body doesn't do numbers: this is its report, and you can't read it. Feeling is the key.

If you want to know how hungry you really are in this moment, you have to stop and take a few minutes to listen carefully to your body. Is that really your stomach announcing its emptiness? Do you need a caloric pick-me-up? Or are you just bored, anxious, annoyed, tired, depressed, and in need of an *emotional* lift?

If there's no false alarm, just *how* hungry are you? Use the scale. If you're at one or two, it's time for a healthy meal. If you're squarely on one, be careful. When you're ravenous, you're more likely to eat anything, because when the body truly is in need it's not picky. Also, if you have blood sugar problems, letting yourself get desperately hungry could cause a low blood sugar crash, which makes you feel lousy in general but also makes you crave sugary carbohydrates.

Frankly, you should flat-out avoid hunger one. It's just too powerful a condition! If you're often finding yourself here, you really should rework your daily plans so you're able to eat earlier.

Ideally, your true hunger will be in the two or three range. If it's at four, you're not really hungry. Bear in mind that the body takes between three to four hours to digest a normal meal. So if you ate only a couple of hours ago and feel hungry, it's likely you aren't. It's quite possible you're actually thirsty. Eating is such a ubiquitous activity that we often misinterpret thirst as hunger.

Water, Water Everywhere

When you feel the kinda-sorta-maybe hunger-ish impulse, try drinking a glass of water; a long, tall glass will soothe many "hunger" pangs promptly. That's because water is a natural appetite suppressant. Studies have shown that 37 percent of Americans have a thirst mechanism that is so weak, they often mistake thirst for hunger. So get out there and get hydrated!

First, water metabolizes fat. Yep, if you enough drink water you can lose weight. And if you drink cold water, you have a chance to burn approximately seventy extra calories a day. There is also a correlation between water intake and fat deposits; generally, when there's more water, there's less fat.

Water makes up about 80 percent of the body's mass. It's essential to keeping physiological systems running efficiently, including digestion, oxygen circulation, cognition, and maintenance of the body's cooling system. Fresh water must come in a steady supply to keep the body in prime functioning form. Water keeps the colon hydrated, which makes pooping a great deal easier. Remember, more pooping, more weight loss.

The average person needs about two liters of water per day. Note that I said *water*, not liquids! Many beverages, particularly soft and alcoholic ones, actually steal tremendous amounts of water from the body. If you've been consuming a few Cokes or after-work drinks out of habit, it's likely you aren't drinking enough water to compensate.

And the lack of water has immediate, observable effects. It is the most common trigger of daytime fatigue. A mere 2 percent drop in water volume can cause fuzzy short-term memory, trouble with basic math, and fragmented concentration. Conversely, proper hydration can reduce the effects of many common ailments, including headaches, fatigue, and joint pain.

A well-hydrated body has a higher level of oxygen in the bloodstream than a dehydrated body. The more available oxygen, the more fat the body can burn for energy; without sufficient oxygen the body will not utilize stored fat efficiently. And of course, more oxygen means more energy; ask any athlete!

Does that water taste any better yet?

Take your water intake seriously. Have some with every meal and a glass or two in between. You're making your body a more efficient metabolic factory, and the task of cutting out calories will be that much less complicated.

If you're still groaning, remember that sparkling water is a legitimate alternative. And it's just as refreshing as any other carbonated beverage. Try it: crack open a bottle of your favorite brand on a hot day; would you describe your first sip as bland? I didn't think so.

No Kidding, I'm Really Still Hungry, AND Hydrated!

Fine, then please, eat some more. But don't abandon that body awareness. Eating doesn't satisfy your feeling of hunger immediately. Generally speaking, it takes about twenty minutes for your brain to catch up with your stomach and decide that you've eaten enough to stop being hungry. Unfortunately, that signal from the brain is easy to miss. When you're very hungry, when you've got a lot of food in front of you, when it's a favorite food, when you've had a drink or two, when you're enjoying a meal with friends, when you're entertaining for business—your attention isn't on your hunger/fullness level. You're in the moment, bombarded by plenty of cues that say yes to eating long after your stomach has announced that it's had quite enough, thank you.

The best place to hone your awareness of hunger and fullness is at home. I advise taking a break at the halfway point during normal meals and rating hunger right then. If your stomach is still unsatisfied, go ahead and eat more, but with level five—the sweet spot of satisfaction—in mind. Generally, once you're accustomed to stopping at five, you'll discover greater willingness to opt out of dessert and a lot of empty (and unnecessary) calories. You might even decide to not even finish your main course. For people who were raised to always clean their plates, or else, this is a huge step forward.

Just knowing that the hunger/fullness scale goes a full two notches higher than five is another incentive to quit when the body says enough. We all know about the uncomfortable and embarrassing effects of overeating: the unpleasant abdominal pressure and sleepy fatigue, the heartburn, reflux, gas, bloating, diarrhea, and constipation, not to mention the weight gain!

Like most other aspects of my program, I don't expect you to become fanatically aware of this scale. And I don't recommend skipping or delaying meals if your appetite isn't at two or three. Hunger will build up, with intense physical and mental messages, if you don't eat something during a normal mealtime. And by the next, you may well be at the level one extreme, and the calories saved by skipping the first meal will be made up, and then some, at the next. The virtue of not eating because you're at level four could be undone by a later, desperate stop at a drive-through and a dose of fast food. So don't skip those meals, just make them smaller, or turn them into snacks.

I'm Not Hungry, I'm...?

Once you're used to the hunger/fullness scale, it's reasonable to ask what's *really* behind that restlessness that, traditionally, sent you in search of food.

For some of us, the desire to eat is triggered just by the presence of food. If it's there, we eat it. And if a lot of it is there, we eat it all. This is mindless eating—and it's very, very common, even in people who don't have weight issues.

In an experiment that's become famous, psychologist Brian Wansink, author of the fascinating *Mindless Eating,* invited people to see a free movie. Inside the theater, some were given big buckets of stale popcorn; others were given *huge* buckets of stale popcorn. Happy eating, folks!

The researchers took the buckets back when the people left theater. They found that the people who were given the huge buckets actually ate *more* of the popcorn than those given the smaller (but still very large) buckets.

What was going on here? Why would someone eat her way through a huge container of stale, cold popcorn?

Well, when it comes to food and visual cues, size matters! We rely on external cues—such as the size of the serving container—for instruction on how much to eat. Large containers—or large plates full of food—urge us to eat everything in or on them, even when our hunger would be more than satisfied by a smaller portion. Listen to your body? Why do that? After all, a movie theater wouldn't provide those big buckets if there was something wrong with eating that much, right?

And that's the situation, in an extra-large bucket. Visual cues trigger eating, and they often overrule a body's subtle messages. All that food sure looks good in its attractive packaging, and the people who eat it sure look happy (in the ads, anyway). Why should you miss out?

I can't make you turn off your television or close your eyes when you walk through a shopping district that's filled with familiar logos that all announce, "Come and eat!" But try to be mindful of how ads and billboards and other food triggers affect you. There's a lot of quick happiness in those restaurants; you think about the food inside, and when you next pass the restaurant, you want the food. The colors on the cookie box or the bag of chips might evoke happy childhood memories. You know what's going on; intellectually, you may be aware that clever advertising is affecting you. But that doesn't mean it stops working on the gut level.

Then there are the dinners that are spoiled when you pillage the breadbasket before your order arrives. You can plow through hundreds of calories worth of rolls and butter before you've even sipped your soup. Don't just accept this as "the way it is": ask the waiter to remove the basket after you've taken one roll, or request that it never appear.

A lot of mindless eating is of the "because it's there" variety: you need to use your mind to put a stop to it.

Don't Let Your Kids Do Your Thinking

When you have children at home, it's easy to fall into mindless eating and dig into junk food that you bought for your kids. But think it through: your kids don't need to be eating this stuff any more than you do. You're the parent: it's OK to try setting a good example.

With a healthy nutritional IQ, you're better able to understand why and how to make better snack choices. And you can give your kids a head start on healthy eating; perhaps then they'll avoid yo-yo dieting and loss of food control that you're working so hard to overcome.

How Many Calories Do You *Really* Need?

You'll recall from chapter four that basal metabolism rate (BMR) is the number of calories you need each day to maintain your body weight. You can determine your BMR with a fairly simple formula.

If you're woman, multiply your body weight in pounds by ten, or if in kilograms by twenty-two. If you're a man, multiply your body weight in pounds by eleven or by twenty-four if you're using kilograms. (The difference is because men have more muscle than women, lucky bastards!)

Let's imagine that Greta is 155 pounds. So the minimum amount of calories she needs is:

$$155 \text{ pounds} \times 10 = 1{,}550$$

Greta needs 1,550 calories a day. That's the bare minimum number of calories she needs each day just to stay healthy and avoid malnutrition.

About two-thirds of the calories you eat each day keep your heart beating, your lungs breathing, your brain thinking, and your body repair functions operating normally. These functions go on all the time, so you burn calories even when you're sleeping. Another 10 percent or so of your calories go toward keeping your digestive system moving along and metabolizing your food.

So that's about three-quarters of your calories expended, just keeping you alive.

The other 25 percent goes toward physical activity—all the walking and moving around you do in the course of an ordinary day. Any leftover calories will come from that last 25 percent; they will be stored in your body as fat if they're not burned off during your activities.

So, to determine how many calories you need beyond your basal metabolism rate, you must honestly scrutinize your activity level. The formula now become a little more complicated, but it's still quite basic.

First, you need to calculate what's called your lifestyle percentage (L%). This is an estimate of how active you are as a percentage of your BMR. You could do an elaborate study of your daily activity to figure this out, but it's much easier to just use standard estimates based on your lifestyle.

If you lead a sedentary life with not much physical activity (you work at a desk all day and don't exercise), your lifestyle percentage (L%) is near 20 percent of your BMR.

If you're somewhat active (you're on your feet a lot at work), your L% is probably 30 percent of your BMR.

If you're moderately active (you're on your feet all day at work, then you do a lot of housework or gardening), your L% is 40 percent of your BMR.

And if you're very active (you do construction or other active work or exercise hard a couple of hours a day) your L% might touch 50 percent of your BMR.

To figure out how many calories you need each day, add together your BMR and your lifestyle percentage. If you're a 140-pound woman, your BMR is 1,400 calories. If you're also moderately active, your lifestyle percentage is 30 percent of 1,400 calories, or 420 calories. Add the numbers together and you get 1,820 calories. That's the number of calories our imaginary woman needs each day to stay at her current weight and activity level. If you're overweight, your BMR and L% together will keep you at your current weight, even though it's higher than you want.

Of course, these numbers aren't precise, and I certainly wouldn't expect you to measure everything down to the calorie. That would be obsessive and ultimately not too helpful.

As a good rule of thumb, if you're a normal-weight woman who is moderately active, you need about 1,200 to 1,500 calories a day. A normal-weight, moderately active man needs about 2,000 to 2,500 calories a day. If you're at your normal weight and want to stay there, stay at the right number of calories for your activity level. If you're usually moderately active and for some reason become a lot more sedentary, you'll gain weight even if you're still taking in the same number of calories, because you're not burning off as many.

And How Many Calories Can You Cut?

Many of my clients could never understand why they had gotten heavier. They swore they were not eating any more than they ever did. I believed them, most of the time, anyway.

If you recall chapter four, you probably have an explanation for most of these people: life isn't fair, and they're getting older. Since metabolism slows down as adulthood advances, you simply *can't* eat as you did at twenty when you're fifty and avoid weight gain. This is particularly true for women after they reach menopause.

Exercise is the antidote to an aging metabolism. It's not negotiable. But as I'll explain in chapter ten, you can find ways to exercise that don't mean trips to the gym and are easy on your joints.

It comes down to this: if you consume more calories or become less active, you'll gain weight. Eat more *and* become less active, and you'll gain weight rapidly.

Fortunately, this also works in reverse: eat less or exercise more, and you'll lose weight. Eat less *and* exercise more, and you'll lose weight faster. By exercising more, you get the metabolic advantage: muscles burn more energy than fat, even when you're just sitting around. More muscle, more calories burned, more weight loss. And when you get down to a comfortable weight, more toned muscles help you stay there by letting you eat a bit more than you could if you didn't exercise.

Meanwhile, you have to craft a diet you can live with. If you're overweight, probably you need to reduce the number of calories you take in each day. But like other aspects of my program, this one doesn't involve sudden, drastic cuts. We're going to ramp down your portions slowly.

Let's say you are 180 pounds/82 kilograms. You need a minimum of 1,800 calories a day to maintain your weight and around 1,300 to lose weight. You *don't* want to carve 500 calories out of your diet immediately; drastic cuts to your diet aren't healthy, and they usually backfire.

Instead, you could start by decreasing by 100 calories a day in your first week. (Keep in mind that one slice of bread has approximately 100 calories.) Once you've had a week at that plateau, cut another 100 calories out during the second week, and so on, until you've reached 500 fewer calories after five weeks. People who are far above their BMR can ramp down at a sharper angle: for instance, 5,300 calories could be cut to 5,000 in week one, then to 4,500 in week two, for example.

Making smart cuts will be easier when you have a clear sense of two things: what you typically eat during the week and how many calories those foods contain. When you assign numbers to foods you often use, your choices will become easier.

Of course, as chapter two made clear, heavily sugared foods should be primary targets. Anything with refined sugars (doughnuts, cookies, cakes) or simple sugar (basically, anything that is white, except for cauliflower) should be reduced or eliminated. Remember, with less sugar in your diet you will enjoy the varied tastes of other foods all the more.

Next, cut back on anything you drink that isn't water, and replace it with… more water! Buy your San Pellegrino if your tongue needs a little pizzazz, but make sure you drink it.

So, Feel Smarter Yet?

You should. If you allow your body to give you the straight story about hunger and think long enough to develop a realistic vision of your daily caloric needs, you're ready to start putting food on your plate, food that you enjoy. And never forget: *breathing* should be an automatic function. Eating never should be.

Summary

- *Remember the basic fact: the calorie is a unit of measurement for food.*

- *Put hunger on the one-to-seven scale, and learn to distinguish between real and false pangs.*

- *Never skimp on your water ration.*

- *Emotions, dehydration, and mindlessness all play a role in overeating.*

- *Determine your BMR and L% to pin down your daily calorie needs.*

- *Make small cuts to make initial reductions in your daily calorie intake.*

Chapter Six

DESIGNING YOUR OWN ACHIEVABLE DIET

Now you are ready to design your own achievable diet—a new approach to eating that will help you lose weight and keep it off. And most of all, you'll never feel hungry or deprived, because you know what hunger *really* is and isn't.

This chapter will show you how easy it is to count calories and catch the excitement that comes from designing your own diet. Your weight loss will happen naturally, and once you're savvier about portion control and the foods you really love, losing will become progressively easier. You might even find it fun.

Think a moment about how far you've come since you got serious about weight loss! By now:

* You know how much weight you want to lose.

* You've begun to detox from sugar.

* You know your eating personality; you've spotted some blind spots and are hunting for more.

* The scale no longer frightens you, and you know your weight common denominator.

* You've given your Nutritional IQ a boost, and you're much more aware of when you're hungry and when you're not.

That takes you at least a few steps past A. This chapter will help you run through a small, pleasant mouthful of letters.

What's on the Menu?

Let's imagine you're set to reduce your weight by eleven pounds/five kilograms. That's a reasonable goal for starters; in fact, once you reach it, I recommend that you maintain this new weight common denominator for as long as six months before you try to lose more. It's always a good idea to give your body time to adjust to new regimens.

You'll also need time to adjust to a different way of thinking about foods. Remember, there's no food that you must never eat again. But there are some that should be reserved for your weekly free meal, and others that should be eaten sparingly the rest of the week. Then, there are the delicious favorites that can be enjoyed just about whenever the mood strikes. Like my client with her morning pineapple, you'll ramp up your portion of some foods you love and cut back on the portions of others.

3,500 Calories = 1 Pound/Approximately Half a Kilo

Understanding the relationship between calories and your weight is the key to an achievable diet. Remember a few key concepts:

If you eat as many calories (food) as you use, your weight will stay steady.

If you eat more calories (food) than you use, you will gain weight.

If you eat fewer calories (food) than you use, you will lose weight.

It's pretty simple, right? Calories in, calories out: if this sounds like a mantra, good! You really need to keep this basic concept in mind. Remember that weight loss, like many aspects of our lives, is only as complicated as we make it!

To gain one pound of body weight, you need to take in about 3,500 calories more than you will use. You gain weight when your body stores extra calories as fat. To lose one pound of body weight, you need to take in 3,500 calories *less* than you use. You lose weight when calorie intake goes down because your body taps your stored fat for energy.

Three thousand five hundred calories may sound like awful lot, but the key to achieving weight loss is realizing that it's less than it seems. If you consistently cut out 3,500 calories a week, you'll lose about a pound/half a kilogram a week. That doesn't mean starving yourself—and in fact, this much loss might be too fast for most people. But if you're eating the typical Westernized diet, you can easily find five hundred calories a day to cut. Add it up: That's 3,500 for seven days, a pound/half a kilogram a week.

Just one can of soda, for example, has about 150 calories. If you're drinking two a day, that's 300 calories every day that can easily be replaced by sparkling mineral water or plain water—with zero calories. With 300 empty calories removed from your daily intake, you're on track to lose one pound/half a kilogram in about twelve days; that works out to 30 pounds/13.6 kilograms over the course of a year! If you simultaneously increase you activity level, you'll shed the weight even faster.

Remember this: to figure the calories you need to maintain your current weight (yes, yes, I know you want to *lose* weight), simply multiply your weight in pounds by ten or your weight in kilograms by twenty-two.

So if you are 180 pounds, just add a zero: 180 times 10. One thousand eight hundred calories is what you need to eat to keep your weight.

Weight in Pounds x 10 = Approximate Daily Calorie Count

Weight in Kilograms x 22 = Approximate Daily Calorie Count

To lose weight you shoot for a lower number; maybe you can start by shaving off 300 calories each day, which it means you will now make do with 1,500. Those are easy numbers, and this is an easy system that works. Scroll through lists below and start experimenting. This plan is about your body and its unique needs. It's important to know that if you're going on this weight-loss journey with a friend or a partner, your daily intake will probably be different from his or hers, sometimes dramatically so. In order to achieve your goal, you might need 1,500 calories a day, while your partner can shed pounds at 2,200. And that's OK!

No matter who's there to support you, this is your personal journey. And it doesn't take much to stay on the path; walking an extra thirty minutes or taking a little less at lunch can help you stay within your desired caloric range. Don't forget: every small change is one step closer to a trimmer, healthier you.

Of course, you need to make smart choices about where your calories continue to come from. Unfortunately it's possible to manipulate the calorie-in-calorie-out numbers and lose weight—and still be stupid.

I once had a young university student as a client. She knew just enough about calories to tell me that she planned to eat three chocolate bars, at 300 calories each, and then enough french fries each day to bring her to 1,500 calories. At that rate, she figured she'd lose about a pound/half a kilogram a week.

From the look on my face, I'm sure the student thought I was about to call her crazy. Instead, I told her about a diet I'd attempted at her age, the Nutella diet. I ate 1,200 calories' worth of Nutella every day, and I never felt hungry. I lost weight, too. Oh, and within a couple of weeks I thought my liver was about to explode. My body was sending the unmistakable message that it did *not* like being treated so disrespectfully.

Then I explained to the student why losing weight will backfire if one's approach isn't based on good, balanced nutrition. Her proposed diet could lead to some nasty side effects, including diabetes, liver overload, bad skin, and bad breath. Furthermore, there was the question of sustainability: How long would anyone *really* want to subsist on french fries and candy bars (or Nutella) alone?

My university student was a smart girl and caught on right then. Thank heavens.

Confused? Welcome to the Food/Calorie Colors Academy

Let's face it: losing weight is an unnatural process. You may be so fortunate as to never worry about true hunger, but your body doesn't believe it. It always wants to hold on to what it has. Maybe that survivalist mindset has overstayed its welcome, but you won't be rid of it without some planning.

My program is intended to make an unnatural process as pleasurable—and straightforward—as possible. At first glance, all the diet planning might overwhelm you; you're embarking on an entirely new way of life! Shifting out of old, unhealthy behaviors will take time, and adopting a new, healthier regimen takes even more. That's why you need to celebrate every small success along the A-to-Z road. Just as you benefit from shots of adrenaline while you're exercising, you'll have more will and energy for achieving your weight-loss goals if you give yourself regular, justified praise.

But as I mentioned in chapter three, even some Decision Makers want marching orders. "*I* can't figure out what I want to eat," I've been informed more than a few times. "Just *give* me a list of what to eat and what to run away from!"

Admittedly, I think you can do better by taking ownership of big, bad issues that concern your palate and the food it prefers. But I also accept that for some of us, a little bit of boot camp brings the right spirit for the real challenges of sugar detox and reversal of long-standing habits.

So here we go. I present to you a plan for your first three weeks in the *Yes, You Can* program that would pass muster with any nutritionist.

This plan will help you categorize foods by their dietary content and calorie loads. It will give you all the calories and essential vitamins you need. It will clean your body out. It will help you lose an appreciable amount of weight in just a few weeks.

And it's as simple as a stoplight: Green, Yellow, and Red.

Green is for GO. If you want to lose a lot of weight as quickly as possible, you'll eat foods from the Green Light food list almost exclusively. Sugar detoxers can spend a solid two weeks relying on the Green list as they purge. Most of us, though, find one week in Green Light Land to be plenty.

It will take a little discipline to stick to this phase of your regimen, but you can do it. After all, you've got your free day to look forward to. Green foods include vegetables, fruits, some grains, egg whites, chicken breast and legumes for protein, and dairy products such as low-fat yogurt and milk.

Yellow is for GO *with caution*. Yellow Light foods can be eaten up to three times a week. Once you're firmly entrenched in a new dietary regimen, you can eat these foods even more often, perhaps four or five times weekly. But when you start out, remember that yellow stoplights quickly turn red; you can undo good work by eating too much of these foods. Some foods, such as seafood and certain red meats, appear on the yellow list not because they are high in calories but because they contain some harmful chemicals.

Red is for STOP AND THINK. Red Light foods should be eaten once a week at most. So once you've indulged in a Red Light food, STOP for the rest of the week. Really, these are the foods that should be showing up only at your free meal, unless you're making extreme adjustments in other areas of your diet.

You can stick with this tri-color method throughout the weight-loss process; you could stick with it for the rest of your life, for that matter!

Scroll through each week's list and check off your favorite foods, being especially alert to those that make the Green list. Also, observe my shorthand exercise recommendations; we'll be talking much more about exercise in chapter ten, but I want you to have a sense of what you should be trying to burn as you adopt the routine.

Be aware that all the foods listed are to be grilled, steamed, boiled, or raw, *not* fried. Feel free to add one tablespoon of extra-virgin olive oil to the preparation at lunch or dinner, with as many herbs and spices as you fancy. Keep in mind that a tablespoon of olive oil has approximately 120 calories.

THE *YES YOU CAN* RED, YELLOW AND GREEN LISTS

RED FREE MEAL: EAT UNTIL SATISFIED	YELLOW Up to three times a week	GREEN EVERY DAY	PORTION SIZE (GREEN LIST ONLY)
		(DO NOT JUICE)	
		Lettuce	Until satisfied
		Cucumber	Until satisfied
		Cabbage	Until satisfied
		Radish	Until satisfied
		Asian greens	Until satisfied
		Celery	Until satisfied
		Broccoli	Until satisfied
		Zucchini	Until satisfied
		String beans	Until satisfied
		Beetroot	Until satisfied
		Tomato	Until satisfied
		Eggplant	Until satisfied
		Yellow squash	Until satisfied
		Butternut squash	Until satisfied
		Okra	Until satisfied
		Green peppers	Until satisfied
		Red peppers	Until satisfied
		Asparagus	Until satisfied
		Spinach	Until satisfied
		Leeks	Until satisfied
		Pumpkin	Until satisfied
		Turnips	Until satisfied
		Carrots	Until satisfied

		Brussel sprouts	Until satisfied
		Artichoke	Until satisfied
		Cauliflower	Until satisfied
		Parsnips	Until satisfied
		Choose one of the following daily:	
Chicken wing	Venison	Sweet potato	Fist-sized
Chicken leg	Rabbit	Potato	Fist-sized
Turkey leg	Veal	Corn	Fist-sized
Lamb, leg	Filet steak	Avocado	Fist-sized
Lamb, loin chop	(fat trimmed)	Peas	Fist-sized
Lamb, minced	Chicken thigh	Black-eyed peas	Fist-sized
	(fat trimmed)	Chickpeas	Fist-sized
Catfish	Duck breast	Navy beans	Fist-sized
Orange roughy	(fat trimmed)	Kidney beans	Fist-sized
Shark		Pinto beans	Fist-sized
Swordfish	Crab	Lentils	Fist-sized
	Flounder/sole	Red beans	Fist-sized
Bacon	Monkfish	Soy beans	Fist-sized
Ham	Shrimp	Split/dried peas	Fist-sized
Loin chops	Cod	Butter beans	Fist-sized
Pork shoulder	Clams	Lima beans	Fist-sized
Spare ribs	Sea Bass		
Pork belly	Mahi mahi	**Choose two of the following a day:**	
	Perch	Turkey breast	Palm-sized
Corned beef	Lobster	Chicken breast	Palm-sized
Roast beef	Pike	Veal	Palm-sized

Chuck top round	Scallops	Salmon (fresh)	Palm-sized
Skirt steak	Bass	Salmon (canned, in water)	Palm-sized
Flank steak	Mackerel	Tuna (canned, in water)	Palm-sized
Sirloin steak	Abalone	Snapper	Palm-sized
Ground beef (minced)	Halibut	Light ham	Palm-sized
T-bone steak	Sardines (canned)	Tofu	Palm-sized
Brisket	Bluefish	Tempeh	Palm-sized
Porterhouse	Carp		
New York steak	Octopus	**Choose one or a combination of following, daily:**	
Tenderloin	Mussels	Plum	Two pieces/ two cups
Prime rib	Trout	Strawberries	Until satisfied
Rib-eye steak	Tuna (steak)	Apricots	Two pieces/ two cups
		Guava	Two pieces/ two cups
	Veggie burgers	Tangerine	Two pieces/ two cups
	Textured vegetable protein	Peach	Two pieces/ two cups
	Soy milk (one cup)	Cantaloupe	Two pieces/ two cups
	Soy yogurt (one cup)	Raspberries	Two cups
		Papaya	Two pieces/ two cups

		Kiwi	Two pieces/ two cups
		Nectarine	Two pieces/ two cups
		Honeydew melon	Two pieces/ two cups
		Orange	Two pieces/ two cups
		Apple	Two pieces/ two cups
		Pineapple	Two pieces/ two cups
		Blueberries	Two cups
		Cherries	Two cups
		Pear	Two pieces/ two cups
		Banana	Two pieces/ two cups
		Grapes	Two cups
		Pomegranate	Two pieces/ two cups
		Mango	Two cups
		Coconut	Two cups
	Choose one of the following (fist-sized portion):	Choose one of the following for breakfast and lunch:	
White bread	Basmati rice	Whole meal bread	Two pieces
Bagels	White rice	Whole grain bread	Two pieces
English muffins	Jasmine rice	Rye bread	Two pieces
Pikelet	Rice noodles	Sourdough bread	Two pieces

	Couscous	Pumpernickel bread	Two pieces
	Gnocchi		
	Udon noodles	**Choose one of the following, daily, cooked:**	
		Wild rice	Fist-sized
	Two times a week:	Barley	Fist-sized
	Raisins	Brown rice	Fist-sized
	Sultanas	Quinoa	Fist-sized
		Choose two of the following:	
		Dry crackers	
		Rice crackers	
		Corn cakes	
		Rice cakes	
		Choose one of the following, daily:	
ALL high-sugar, low fiber cereals		Rolled oats	Fist-sized
		Porridge	Fist-sized
		Natural muesli	Fist-sized
		Choose one of the following, daily:	
Ice cream	Low-fat custard	Low-fat milk	One cup
Flavored milk		Skim milk	One cup
Whole milk		Low-fat yogurt	One cup
Full-fat yogurt			

		Choose one or combine, daily	Small handful (your hand!)
Salted nuts		Almonds	
		Brazil nuts	
		Cashews	
		Hazelnuts	
		Pistachios	
		Walnuts	
ALL cookies		Poppy seeds	
Milk chocolate		Pumpkin seeds	
Candy		Sesame seeds	
Cake			
Turkish bread		Dark chocolate	Two squares
Fruit juice	Caffeinated tea	Water	Unlimited
Soda pop	Coffee	Sparkling water	Unlimited
Cordials		Herbal tea	Unlimited

What's in My Food?

You're probably used to counting calories from time spent on other weight-loss regimens, or at least flipping through a magazine or two. Since we'll be counting again throughout this program, let's take a little time to break down the food groups and talk about what they deliver in terms of calorie loads.

Vegetables: 101 Ways to Eat

A single serving of a vegetable is generally one cup, cooked or raw as customary for the food. Surprise, surprise: vegetables tend to be lower in calories than meat and seafood. This means you can have larger servings without worrying too much about packing on pounds/kilograms (unless you're drowning them in Hollandaise sauce). Starchier vegetables (such as potatoes, sweet potatoes, avocados, and corn) tend to be higher in calories than green vegetables, and often they're prepared in a fashion that adds plenty of extra calories (think creamed corn and mashed potatoes). Again, bear in mind that you can make key calorie reductions simply by changing the way you prepare certain foods; butter, dairy, and other additives are high in calories, so it's better to use olive oil and herbs for seasoning. If you have the discipline (and the palate), stick to vegetables on the lower end of the caloric scale.

All the calorie counts below represent about seven ounces, or two hundred grams, about a cup measure:

Vegetable	Calories
Arugula	6
Lettuce	10
Cucumber	16
Cabbage	17
Radish	19
Bok choy	20
Celery	23
Broccoli	25
Broccoli rabe	25
Fennel	27
Zucchini	29
Mustard greens	29
String beans	34
Beets	35
Swiss chard	35
Tomato	35
Eggplant	35
Kale	36

Yellow squash	36
Okra	36
Green peppers	38
Chayote	38
Asparagus	40
Spinach	41
Red peppers	46
Jicama	46
Kohlrabi	48
Leeks	48
Collards	49
Pumpkin	49
Turnips	51
Carrots	54
Brussels sprouts	56
Artichoke	64
Cauliflower	64
Butternut squash	94
Sweet potato, medium	103
Parsnips	111
Corn	112
Acorn squash	115
Potato, medium	144
Avocado, medium	227

Fruit

Fruit servings are one cup/two hundred grams/seven ounces, or one medium piece, uncooked. As with vegetables, fruits often are much lower in calories than meats and seafood, which makes them great snacks. Their natural sweetness also can act as a fine substitute when you're detoxing from refined sugars. Be aware of the portion sizes, however; sugar is still sugar. If you're detoxing, you might want to hold your fruit intake to one cup a day.

Fruit	Portion	Calories
Apricot	1 medium	17
Plum	1 medium	30
Guava	1 medium	37
Tangerine	1 medium	40
Grapefruit	½ medium	44
Watermelon	1 cup/200 g	46
Figs, fresh	1 large	47
Strawberries	1 cup/200 g	49
Peach	1 medium	51
Cantaloupe	1 cup/200 g	54
Raspberries	1 cup/200 g	54
Papaya	1 medium	55
Kiwi	1 medium	56
Nectarine	1 medium	57
Honeydew melon	1 cup/200 g	61
Orange	1 medium	62
Blackberries	1 cup/200 g	62
Apple	1 medium	72
Pineapple, fresh	1 cup/200 g	74
Blueberries	1 cup/200 g	84
Cherries	1 cup/200 g	87
Pear	1 medium	96
Grapes	1 cup/200 g	104
Banana	1 medium	105
Mango	1 medium	135
Pineapple, canned	1 cup/200 g	149
Pomegranate	1 medium	234
Coconut	1 cup/200 g	283
Raisins	1 cup/200 g	498

Tofu, Beans, and Legumes

This is an important group if you're serious about weight loss and prefer a vegetarian approach. Tofu is loaded with protein, which is why it shows up so often in vegan and vegetarian recipes; it plays the role beef does for many carnivores. Beans are also protein rich. While these foods are not complete proteins, by combining them with other foods (such as good ol' beans and rice), you can easily receive sufficient protein, as well as plenty of fiber and other goodness.

Food	Portion	Calories
Black beans	½ cup/125 g	105
French beans	1 cup/177 g	228
Great Northern	½ cup/121 g	110
Kidney beans	1 cup/256 g	215
Pinto beans	1 cup/171 g	243
Refried beans	1 cup/252 g	237
Chickpeas	1 cup/240 g	286
Lentils	1 cup/198 g	115
Firm tofu	1 cup/252 g	176
Tempeh	1 cup/166 g	320

Grains

A single serving of a grain is one cup/two hundred grams/seven ounces cooked. Generally, these foods are more caloric than fruits and veggies, while still coming in below animal products. As with vegetables, preparation is key: stick to recipes that rely more on spices and olive oil, and try to avoid white flour and white rice when possible.

Grain	Calories
Bulgur	151

Buckwheat	155
Wild rice	166
Whole-wheat pasta	174
Basmati rice	179
Barley	193
White rice	205
Millet	207
Brown rice	216
Semolina pasta	221
Quinoa	222
Amaranth	251
Jasmine rice	280

Meat

One rule to keep in mind regarding meat: the cuts that are highest in fat also are highest in calories. Beef lovers who enjoy filet mignon can make reductions simply by choosing lean or extra-lean cuts. Generally, a lean cut of beef has less than ten grams of fat per one one-hundred-gram serving; an extra-lean cut has about five grams of fat.

All the servings listed below are cooked and represent 100 grams, or about 3.5 ounces. That's a piece of meat about the size of a pack of cards; probably this is less than you're accustomed to, and *certainly* it's less than the slabs served in most restaurants!

Meat	*Calories*
Beef	
Corned beef	160
Roast beef	184
London broil	190
Bottom-round steak	206
Tri-tip roast	235
Bottom-round roast	242

Chuck steak	245
Top round	248
Skirt steak	249
Flank steak	266
Sirloin steak	300
Filet mignon	302
Ground, 20% fat	308
T-bone steak	318
Brisket	326
Porterhouse steak	336
Chuck roast	342
Club steak (NY steak)	365
Tenderloin	366
Prime rib	381
Rib eye steak	404

Game

Venison	118
Snake	124
Kangaroo	138
Wild boar	181
Buffalo	200
Rabbit	227
Alligator	253
Veal	261

Lamb

Leg	162
Loin chop	183
Ground	198
Stew meat	252

Poultry

Chicken egg	78

Chicken breast	142
Chicken thigh	153
Turkey breast	153
Emu	160
Ostrich	175
Duck breast	300
Chicken wing	99
Chicken leg	181
Turkey leg	192

Pork

Bacon	172
Canadian bacon	172
Ham	188
Tenderloin	195
Pork chops, loin	272
Pork shoulder	304
Spare ribs, back	415
Pork belly	588

Seafood

These portions of seafood are about three and a half ounces, or 114 grams each. Cold-water ocean fish are generally oilier and higher in calories because they contain more omega-3 fatty acids. So be smart: keep them in your diet.

Ocean fish actually could be marketed exclusively as beauty agents. The oils in these fish are extremely beneficial to your skin's health. They help protect against UV radiation, which ages skin and contributes greatly to the growing risk of skin cancer among many world populations. Chemicals call MMPs are linked both to the cancer and wrinkles, but there's hard evidence demonstrating fish oil's ability to restrict the production of MMPs.

Also, those fish oils are terrific for keeping business regular in the colon. They keep the colon hydrated and make it a great deal easier for you to keep your pooping routine as regular as the sunrise. This, too, can reduce your cancer risk down the road, but in the meantime, don't forget that more pooping means more weight loss. There's no need to reach for laxatives (as if there were *anything* normal about putting a normal human function into hyperdrive); sensible nutrition is all you need. I can't emphasize it enough: a healthy, daily poop should make it onto everyone's A-to-Z weight-loss list.

So don't skimp on the salmon. If you love to eat it with a squeeze of lemon, then stick with it throughout the *Yes, You Can* process. There's room for 233 calories of this super food in everyone's diet.

Seafood	*Calories*
Crab	60
Oysters	76
Squid	104
Monkfish	109
Shrimp	112
Tilapia	113
Cod	120
Mahimahi	120
Perch	120
Lobster	120
Pike	121
Haddock	127
Scallops	127
Flounder/sole	130
Sea bass	140
Red snapper	145
Salmon, canned	157
Halibut	159
Bass	165
Clams	168

Bluefish	180
Carp	184
Octopus	185
Mussels	195
Tuna, fresh	208
Tuna, canned in oil	211
Tuna, canned in water	132
Abalone	215
Trout	216
Mullet	218
Salmon, fresh	233
Pompano	239
Mackerel	266
Sardines, canned in oil	310
Orange roughy	118
Shark	148
Catfish	172
Swordfish	176

Ahem, about That Processed Crap

So you've scanned these lists of healthy, recommended foods. But human nature being what it is, I'm guessing that you haven't seen the numbers that *really* interest you. There's a free meal in your immediate future, and while I hope you believe me when I tell you it's OK to eat absolutely anything, it's natural to ask: just how many calories do those sugary and fatty foods pack?

I don't have the space—or the stomach—to provide anything like a comprehensive list. But as an exercise in contrast, have a look at how some of our old favorites stack up against the foods listed above, foods that should be the foundation of your new eating regimen.

The calorie loads here shouldn't be too surprising, with obesity rates climbing as they have in recent years. And of course, who makes these foods and how they prepare them affects the calorie loads. The figures below are probably closer to averages than exact calorie numbers (I mean, you don't use a ruler to measure out your one-eighth of a pie. Do you?).

Food	Calories
French fries, small	275
3 ounces (85 grams):	
Blueberry pie, one slice	360
Chocolate cake, 2.5 ounces	235
(71 grams)	
Jelly doughnut	210
Cream-filled doughnut	250
Chocolate doughnut	310
Hot dog and bun	245
3 ounces (100 grams)	
5 chicken nuggets	280
½ cup vanilla ice cream	270
3½ ounces (100 grams)	
Potato chips, 1 ounce	140
(28 grams)	
Barbecue chips, 7 ounces	972
(198 grams)[2]	
Pepperoni pizza, one slice	181
2.5 ounces (71 grams)	

Alcohol

---

2 I included two servings of potato chips to illustrate the absurdity of the serving sizes listed on food packages. An ounce of potato chips has fewer calories than a serving of salmon, but when was the last time you ate *one ounce* of chips? How many times have you made short work of a full seven-ounce bag? Apply the same principle to the servings of fries, ice cream, and other goodies, and voila, the relationship between these foods and expanding waistlines is easy to see.

Let's have some more plain talk. Alcohol isn't for everyone, of course; plenty of my friends have never much cared for it. But I'd have to say that they're in a minority. Since we've already admitted that this weight-loss process requires hard work, it's quite understandable if you feel like you deserve a tall cold one at the end of your day. By all means, I say, enjoy one. But do it responsibly. Of course that means you shouldn't be driving, but it also means that you should be aware of two things: cocktails can contain a lot of sugar (hello, detoxers! Don't let that info slip past your radar), and not all adult beverages are the same, calorically speaking.

You've probably heard that moderate portions of alcohol seem to have beneficial health effects. Red wine's press clippings have been favorable, and you can find plenty of people (outside of bars) who will speak up for the health benefits of beer, scotch, and other spirits. Moderate consumption of spirits seems to be good news for the heart, but evidence suggests that overall it promotes longevity and protects against other health threats, such as gallstones and—believe it or not—diabetes.

Hooray to all of that. But we're still counting up calories, and there are choices for you here, too. Generally, the purer the spirit, the lower the calorie load. Drinking your scotch (or gin, vodka, or even tequila) neat delivers plenty of bang for the buck for a bargain: most of these drinks deliver between 95 and 120 calories for a 1.5-ounce pour, which is what you'll typically receive when you order a single shot in a bar or restaurant.

Wine is also a good choice; red, white, rose, and sparkling wines all typically deliver around 120 to 125 calories per 5-ounce glass. Light beers typically come in around 100 calories per 12 ounces/340 grams. Generally, the lighter the beer's color, the less caloric it is: pilsners tend to be less caloric than ales and stouts.

But just as heavy sauces can ruin a serving of steamed broccoli, you can load your drink up with calories by adding mixers: fruit juices, soft drinks, margarita mixers, daiquiri blends, milk, and cream. A 5-ounce/141-gram white russian made with whole milk could carry around 300 calories, and a 12-ounce /340-gram pina colada could top 350.

You don't have to skip Friday happy hour even if you're detoxing from sugar. But bear in mind that when it comes to drinking, there's a good argument for taking your favorite spirit straight, with no chasers or mixers!

Adding Up the Day's Calories

Now, let's integrate all this information. Make a list of your every-single-day-or-you-get-cranky foods and look up the calorie count for a recommended portion of each. Then, add up the calories based on your *usual* portion. You soon will figure out where at least some of your weight gain comes from.

Too difficult? Nah, after you do it few times (probably five) you will get into the groove. It will become like checking the tag price on a dress and deciding if you can afford it or not.

When I first start discussing calories with my weight-loss clients, I ask them to estimate how many calories there are in foods they eat regularly, such as slice of whole wheat bread, a medium apple, or a baked chicken leg; then I ask how many of those calories they think come from carbs, protein, and fat. Of course, they're often way off.

So then we undertake a review of calorie counts and portion sizes. It's a lot of information up front, but it really helps clients to understand how quickly calories can add up if there is no awareness of portion standards.

You'll want to compile your own list and breakdown of your regular foods. Below is a typical list:

1 medium glass orange juice = 100 calories

1 cup whole milk = 150 calories

1 cup breakfast cereal = 170 calories

1 can soda = 145 calories

1 slice whole grain bread = 100 calories

1 tablespoon mayonnaise = 60 calories

3 ounces (85 grams) sliced ham = 150 calories

1 medium baked potato = 170 calories

6 ounces (175 grams) french fries = 550 calories

1 medium apple = 100 calories

1 cup broccoli with cream sauce = 60 calories

1 quarter-pound fast-food burger = 410 calories

1 baked chicken leg and thigh = 190 calories

5 chocolate chip cookies = 250 calories

1 1.5-ounce (42-gram) chocolate bar = 210 calories

1 teaspoon sugar = 15 calories

Once you've written an *honest* list of your own typical daily consumption, pay careful attention to the calorie amounts and portion sizes on any packaged food you eat. Make use of the lists in this book, and keep tabs on your diet choices when you're on the go by using free phone apps like Lose It!, MyFitnessPal and MyNetDiary. Web sites such as www.my-calorie-counter.com, www.mayoclinic.com, and www.livestrong.com/thedailyplate can provide details not just for basic foods but individual brands as well. For those of you who like the heft of a book, *Bowes and Church's Food Values of Portions Commonly Used* should always be within reach.

You're going to make very simple changes that will help you cut back on calories while still getting plenty of good food to eat. You have several different ways to do this:

* You can cut back on the portion size of high-calorie foods (the portion will be considerably smaller than what you used to eat). Take a tip from a friend of mine, who likes to say, "You know what a lower-calorie sandwich is? A half a sandwich!"

* You can eat the same portion of a high-calorie food, but you eat it just once a week.

* You can substitute a lower-calorie food (and put more food on your plate).

* You can cut back on both high-calorie foods and portion size and add plenty of low-calorie salad, veggies, poultry, fish, and fruits (adding much more food to your plate!).

* You can avoid alcoholic drinks with sugary mixers.

* You can drink sparkling water or plain water instead of sugary canned sodas.

I suggest that you mix and match these methods. When you begin the *Yes, You Can* program, you can start by reducing your portion of T-bone steak and compensating with salad; or have as big a portion of steak as you want just once a week; or stick with the smaller steak and substitute sautéed zucchini (or spinach, salad, asparagus, or broccoli) for french fries; or expand your food horizons and have something new instead of the steak. Or just eat as you normally do and have one light beer instead of two.

You can even make progress simply by changing the order of your dinner courses. Eating some salad before the main course, for instance, is a great way to get a variety of fresh veggies while also assuaging hunger pangs that might lead to overeating.

Varying your methods will introduce you to new, high-nutrition, and low-calorie foods and keep you from getting bored. Meanwhile, your liver will be very appreciative if you cut back on alcohol or switch over to sparkling water or plain water or diluted fruit juice (one-quarter juice and three-quarters water on a cup portion).

If your goal is to lose a modest amount of weight—you want to look leaner or drop down one dress size—mixing and matching your methods is a very effective approach. Even though you've probably been eating quite well, you'll be eating better this way. You'll achieve the weight loss you want without dramatic restrictions.

You'll also steer clear of crash diets that force your body to shed weight at an unnatural, unsustainable speed; they're called "crash" diets for a reason. Crash enthusiasts don't much discuss the second crash—of your ego—that usually follows the diet part. After eating, let's say, only meat for a week, you bite into your first banana and that's probably it. Game over. You'll bloat back to your previous size in no time flat. After eating nothing but protein for that one week, your body will be starved for sugars; it will be in full-on, cave woman emergency mode. So the carb and sugar energy your body receives after being starved will be reserved, as fat. Where? Wherever you don't want to see it, most likely!

Switching to a twenty-first-century century metaphor, a crash diet is like paying exorbitant rent on a house that isn't yours. With this program, you'll make investments that make long-term sense. You'll maintain your "house"—your body—as you would a home that you planned to enjoy and keep for the rest of your life.

Beware the Halo Effect

Remember, we're not always rational about this food business. Many of us can fall prey to the belief that somehow adding salad or vegetables to our plate makes everything else near it magically drop in calories and improve in nutrition. If you have a big serving of pork belly, adding a serving of string beans to your plate does not reduce the number of calories in the pork belly! The only way to cut the calories in a meaningful way is to cut the portion size of the pork belly.

If you decide to have shrimp for supper, you'll be getting about 118 calories—but only if you prepare the shrimp very simply. Deep-frying them in batter might not remove the halo effect of buying low-cal raw shrimp, but it sure will make your calorie count jump. Bake or grill the shrimp with tomatoes and feta cheese; the calories increase less dramatically, and you still have a very satisfying dish. It's even better if you cook it "clean" by putting it on the grill adorned just with some spices and herbs.

Carbs—Fats—Proteins

There are three different kinds of energy that you put into your body: carbs, fats, and proteins. Your body burns energy (calories!) in this order:
1. Carbs
2. Fats
3. Proteins

Just as a car engine needs regular fuel, you need carbs to undertake your activities. As Duke University Medical Center's Eric Westman, MD, MHS, explains it, "We think of carbs as the nutrient that's used first." A few hours after eating, you use carbs for energy and store the excess calories as fat.

Fat comes next. *If your body doesn't have any carbs to burn, it will run on fat. That's how you lose weight.*

But don't turn to Atkins just yet! According to an article from the Harvard School of Public Health, a yearlong study, published in 2007 in the *Journal of the American Medical Association*, followed overweight, premenopausal women on four diets. The women steadily lost weight for the first six months, with the most rapid weight loss occurring among the Atkins dieters. But after six months, *most of the women started to regain weight.* Why? Because total carb banishment is next to impossible; you can forgo the bagels for a while, but eventually (especially if you're stressed), you'll give in to a craving. Or two. You're a cave woman again, and back to those fattening habits!

Reinvention of the Food Pyramid

So what's the bottom line? Your body and brain need carbs for health and balance. The evidence is clear that excess protein, especially when it's delivered in red meat, causes problems with the heart, kidneys, and more. You're much better off with sensibly apportioned amounts of complex carbs, such as whole grains, fruits, and vegetables, for breakfast and lunch.

I'm sure you remember that pyramid they showed you back in health class (never mind if you can't remember the individual building blocks). Well, now I want you to flip that pyramid upside down. Imagine that its wide base is now on top: it represents your first—and biggest—meal of the day. The meals you eat subsequently will each be a little smaller; there can be several of them if they're small, but none will be bigger than the first. By evening, when you're relaxing at home, you'll be satisfied with your smallest meal of the day.

Breakfast: You should come out of breakfast feeling satisfied, so eat carbs! Take a slice of whole-grain bread (check the labels to make sure it has less than 1 percent fat) with a teaspoon of honey, a small sliced banana, or a dollop of jam. Stay away from sugary cereals, but experiment with other kinds of carbs, both savory and lightly sweetened. A small piece of fruit is always a good choice. Have a coffee if you like, as long as it doesn't have milk, and sweeten it with stevia rather than sugar or artificial sweeteners. Drink as much herbal tea as you want.

Then, after you've enjoyed the meal, think of ways to add extra movement to your day.

Midmorning: It's important to eat a little something before traditional "lunch" time. Why? If you don't, you'll get hungry—probably too hungry— later. This is a good time for a little boost. Try greek yogurt, ten almonds, or a piece of fruit.

Lunch: Vegetables in any form (except juiced)! Make minestrone soup; bake veggies with a sprinkle of cheese; steam them with lemon and plenty of herbs; sauté your favorites with a tablespoon of olive oil and garlic; throw raw carrots into your purse (and don't forget about them!). Add some cottage cheese, black beans, or steamed fish to the portion of vegetables.

Midafternoon: If you've already had yogurt for your morning snack, go for the white of a hardboiled egg or raw veggies with a tablespoon of hummus. Be mindful of portions. Don't use your celery stick like a scooper after every single bite. Instead, spread a thin layer of hummus on top of the stalk. You'll get the same flavor without the extra calories.

3 p.m.: This is the deadline for eating carbs. By this point of the day, you've certainly had your share.

Dinner: You should sit down to this last meal in the hunger-three zone, perhaps even four: you want some food but you aren't *starving*. Thank yourself for taking proactive steps to fill your body with good, clean energy.

* If you are vegan or vegetarian, refer to the Green list and use your imagination to prepare your favorite meal.

* Meat eaters have a choice of protein, such as fish (once or twice a week), chicken breast, or once a week an iron-rich cut of red meat.

* Go for vegetables in any combination: get creative! There are plenty of options online from foodandwine.com, allrecipes.com, and dozens of other sites. YouTube offers plenty of how-to cooking videos, and encyclopedic but approachable manuals like Mark Bittman's *How to Cook Everything* can help you find ideas to keep your dinners fresh and inventive.

Night: If you like, eat two squares of 70 to 85 percent pure chocolate. Be sure to stick with to this limit; you know how easy it is to go down that binging road! Ask supportive friends or family to help keep your appetite in check. Be proactive, and skip this last nibble if the temptation to over-indulge seems overpowering.

Reality Talk

I can already hear you saying, "It's so difficult to eat in the morning. I only have time to shower and get to the train." It's also hard to eat a large breakfast if you've always saved your biggest meal for nighttime. Some people who are used to big meals after dark wake up still feeling full from yesterday's dinner. Who wants to start with a big breakfast in that condition?

I understand. But as you probably have noticed by now, I don't think you can lose your weight and remain slender without changing some deeply ingrained habits. Eating the biggest meal first may require you to wake up earlier, and certainly it will require you to adjust your conception of what dinner is (unless it's a free meal). But really, these are changes you are more than capable of making.

I like to compare the change to a breakfast-first regimen to recovering from jet lag. As international travelers know only too well, jet lag can be a real beast; if you don't have a plan for overcoming the effects, they can last for days. But if you're disciplined, you try to stay awake as long as you can on that first day. You take melatonin, you do everything you can to fall asleep when everyone else is and not at two in the afternoon. The first day is hard, but if you stick to a plan, the worst of the jet lag's effects end after twenty-four hours.

It can be the same with a change to morning eating from night eating. The first dinner will be a big challenge; you'll want to keep it small, even though your stomach will tell you it's in serious need. I recommend filling up on vegetables until the light calorie loads of dinner feel normal, or something like normal.

Once you're accustomed to the new schedule, you will wake up hungry and eager to eat a satisfying breakfast of carbs and protein. And you'll derive as much satisfaction from it as any dinner. It's a fundamental—but simple—shift in orientation. Takes effort? Of course. Possible? Absolutely it is.

Clean: The Best Way to Cook your Food

"Eat clean, stay lean!" is a common expression used by people who exercise and look after their health and their appearance. If you don't consider yourself much of a cook, "clean food," and this program are for you.

"Clean food" is prepared with no butter, no cream, and no elaborate sauces. All you need to do is steam, grill, or boil your food, and then you can add any herbs you'd like. Basil, parsley, garlic, cumin, onions, rosemary, and other spices, either fresh or powdered, add tremendous amounts of flavor without weighing food down with extra calories.

Your food remains clean even if you add that spoonful of extra virgin olive oil (raw only, never cooked) or a teaspoon of avocado as a garnish at each meal.

You can enjoy chicken, seafood, and other big-ticket nutrition items more often in a clean state. If you're a dedicated carnivore, you should become a fan of clean.

Now, if you're still frightened by the idea of cooking anything, let me make it simple. Take a piece of meat, fish, chicken, whatever, and hold it over an open flame. When you think it's done, remove it. Then eat it. If you want to be a little more sophisticated (and still close to the clean ideal), spray a little olive oil on a pan, throw the protein on with vegetables, and cook until it looks done. No thinking required.

There you go: cooking instructions in one paragraph. Now you have no more excuses!

Your Weekly Free Meal, What Is It?

All right, you've planned out a strategy for six good days of eating with an eye toward weight loss. You're careful with Red list foods and getting great nutrition from the Yellow and Green lists. Now, you have a reward for your diligence and creativity. It's time for your free meal.

As I stated in this book's introduction, this isn't about falling off the wagon, being bad, cheating, feeling guilty, losing control, or any other self-defeating concept.

Your free meal is exactly that: free. In controlled situations, which you have planned for, it should always be a pleasure to eat a delicious meal without concern for calories or your waistline. Whether you're making good on a Sunday dinner tradition or hosting a blowout brunch (with bloody marys) for friends, your efforts of the other six days earn you one meal without restrictions.

You will *not* put back on the weight you've been losing during the rest of the week. So be religious about observing this weekly indulgence. You want your body to get used to digesting and burning this heavy meal. Your mind and emotions will appreciate this short but regular vacation from routine.

You may be surprised to discover, however, that after a few months in this program, even your free days might undergo some voluntary changes. Yes, maybe you'll still go for the double-stuffed pepperoni pizza or the giant burger and fries. But you might have developed a taste for broiled shrimp, broccoli with olive oil and hot pepper flakes, and baked potatoes (with a big slab of cake for dessert!). Whatever you choose, you'll enjoy the food all the more because the meal truly will be a special occasion.

Yes, maybe I learned about this concept from a narcissistic bodybuilder, but generations of French and Italian women relied on it to stay slim throughout their lives, too.

Wait! Don't Leave Me Alone to Plan the Menu!

If you're feeling overwhelmed, I understand. You are changing not just how you eat but how you live.

So go back and read through this chapter until you've got it. If it's still unclear, read through it again. A change of mindset and habit will take time and repetition. And as I told you in chapter one, you probably already know a great deal about what you should be eating during the week and what you shouldn't.

But there may be other dynamics hanging you up. We'll explore some possible reasons for being stuck in the next two chapters.

Summary

- *Becoming aware of the caloric content of foods as well as how many calories you need to maintain your weight is key to weight loss. Make a list of your favorite foods from the Red, Yellow, and Green Lists.*

- *A simple way to approach your weight loss in the beginning is to stick with foods on the Green Light list, eating Yellow List foods for two or three times a week and Red Light foods once a week.*

- *Count calories by being aware of portion sizes of your favorite foods and other selections from the Green, Yellow, and Red Lists.*

- *It is important to understand portion sizes when developing a healthier eating plan. Figure out the portion sizes for the foods you eat the most.*

- *Slowly replace high-calorie, unhealthy foods with healthier options.*

- *It's important to eat varied, nutritionally rich foods rather than limiting yourself to one or two foods.*

- *Carbs are not out of your life, but eat most of them for breakfast. Decrease your portion sizes until three p.m., when the carb train stops.*

- *Eat clean and stay lean.*

- *Eat a free meal once a week during which you don't worry at all about calories and/or portion sizes.*

Chapter Seven

WEIGHT LOSS SUCCESS AND SABOTAGE

S abotage? That's right. Our culture of abundance has sabotaged many weight-loss attempts. So has peer pressure. Family dynamics have sunk their share.

You might believe you can skip this chapter. After all, you have friends and family who are completely supportive. You're aware of the media campaigns and the subtle messages. You can't be tricked into eating junk food.

Well, if it's true, more power to you. But watch for blind spots. You have made many intimate relationships through the years, and a great many people have influenced you. Maybe your weight gain had nothing to do with anyone else—many of us are our own worst enemies, after all. But look closer. Eating is a factor in everyone's personal life, and the connection between food and emotions is very, very strong. Almost every client I've had ultimately discovered some person or situation that, consciously or not, aided and abetted his or her weight gain and sabotaged efforts to reverse it. External factors often help us fall off the weight-loss wagon.

Whether you've adopted the A-to-Z arrangement or not, your weight-loss attempt is a journey. Sometimes you'll stall; other times you'll relapse. You are only human, after all. The people who have sabotaged you are human, too, of course; I'm not suggesting that you need to purge your social calendar or disown your family. But you will need to increase your awareness of the emotional traps that have helped you to stay overweight. You can still love the people who have made things difficult for you, but you will have to exercise greater control over your relationships with them.

You can't change your lifestyle and eating habits in a vacuum, which is why many diet programs, however sound, are in trouble from the start. They don't acknowledge the challenges that have nothing to do with calorie counts and everything to do with our state of mind, our families and friendships. But this program is designed to meet these challenges head-on; when I told you that weight loss is a lifestyle change, I really meant it!

The Power of Your Internal Dialogue

Before you prepare to handle the world at large, you must take on your internal dialogue.

When it comes to losing weight, the most potent "enemy" you have to fight might be...*you*!

When you're too heavy, it's easy to blame practically any trouble on your weight. The extra pounds ruin everything. "If only I could slim down, all my problems would be solved" is a statement I've heard many times.

It's not fair, but this attitude is totally understandable. Your weight is something *you* control, and the situations in your life may be beyond your control. It's natural to focus on one circumstance you can control and believe it contains the key to handling others. If you were thinner, more people would like you. You'd get more respect at your job. It would be easier to find the partner you deserve. And so on.

For all the power of this negative internal dialogue, it remains a quiet affair. It doesn't hold up long under scrutiny. If you could record it as you would a phone conversation between two friends, you'd collapse in laughter or shame. The delusions that persist! That are taken so seriously! And all that magical thinking! If you are overweight, I suspect the following trains of thought may look familiar:

"I am hungry, but I am not going to have that doughnut. No. *No.* Oh well, just a bite. Who cares? I deserve it. Who wants to be a skinny bitch anyway? Yum, that tastes good. Oh damn, I ate it. What is *wrong* with me? Why did I *do* that? Damn, that's it. Nothing else for me this week besides salad. I've ruined everything. No more sugar until Monday."

You see the method here? Set up a temptation. Frame it in a "good girl or bad girl" context. Fall for the temptation and open the floodgates of recrimination, self-loathing, and every possible harsh judgment. When you're that bad, how can you feel any compassion for yourself? How can you ever become your own advocate?

Inside the Mind of a Slender Person

Remember in chapter one when we talked about the myth of the skinny person who is blessed by the metabolic gods? It dies hard. But now that you're tasked with changing your internal dialogue, you have to kill this myth dead. No one is slender without doing a few things right.

To prove this, in recent years I've been interviewing people from different backgrounds, educational levels, weights, and ages who had just one thing in common: a slim and toned body. I asked all of them the same questions: When you see something you really would like to eat but you know it will weigh you down, how do you stop? What do you tell yourself? Here are a few of their answers:

* Not now. I can eat it later. I better get the hell out of here so I don't see it or think about it.

* If I eat it, it'll make me feel good for a minute, but then I will feel so bad a few minutes later. I don't want that feeling.

* Eating this will make me fat.

* This will go straight on my ass, right here!

* What's more important? A few minutes of eating pleasure or the ongoing pleasure of looking hot?

Interesting comments, are they not? There's some mild finger-wagging going on here, but a lot more delayed gratification that's based on self-respect. They know they value their health and shape more than any food craving, and that knowledge is enough to keep them out of trouble.

I've also gotten on record people who couldn't resist food temptations. When they encountered a high-calorie food and gave into the craving, their dialogues—or the lack of them—provide a striking contrast to the abstainers':

* All I hear is silence. It's sort of like entering a dark corridor where nobody can see me and all this is in my own mind! It is a strange feeling, silence.

* Oh, whatever, I am hungry.

* I will start to eat better tomorrow.

* Starting Monday, I will never touch a cookie ever again, I will be so strict. I will lose my weight by the beginning of summer.

* I had such a horrible day that a piece of cake will make me feel better. Besides, it is not going to make me fat.

What's different? Notice that these dialogues don't start out nasty: that comes later. But they all presume that what happens now *doesn't matter*. It will be fixed by better behavior later on (no, it won't). No one decision contributes to weight gain (yes, it does, if it's part of a standing pattern). Life is pretty lousy anyway. Or just silence: Don't you get the sense that the person in the dark hall was walking headlong into a trap?

In each case, the person couldn't summon a compelling reason to help him- or herself. So they all gave in and invited a follow-up harangue about weakness, losing at life, being worse than other people.

You can make the best A-to-Z plan yet known to humankind. But it will never get off the drawing board if you can't make your internal dialogue calm, gentle, rational, and forgiving.

Baby Steps

Your internal dialogue is no less than an affirmation of your ability to effect changes in your life. It's not just some mantra. It should make you feel good about you and act as a reminder that no matter what happens, or whom you talk to, you've got a friend. Internal dialogue harnesses the same willpower you use when you stop yourself from buying a pair of shoes you can't afford.

I think it always helps to have some fun. Sometimes the best way to reduce the pressure to be good, or bad, is to laugh about it. You're not brokering world peace; it's just food, after all!

My client Charlotte came up with a great method for setting a good internal tone:

A few days after I started the program, I left work with a craving for my old favorite, extra-large french fries. I knew it was trouble, but I had just enough control to stop and listen to my internal dialogue, as if I were eavesdropping instead of creating it. It was verbal Ping-Pong: "Great! I'll get fries and eat them all driving home." "No, I shouldn't. I went to Diana so I could stop buying these damn fries." "One time! It's OK, we'll make this the free day!" "Stop! I'm a professional physiotherapist! I know what's going on. This is a stupid conversation!" "But I'm hungry!" "OK, then I'll eat a banana. I'll eat two!"

In the end, I ate the bananas and they filled me up. I was able to kind of jump outside the dialogue and see what was funny about it. And I felt great about doing the right thing.

You are not remaking your world in seven days. You're just making a few positive changes, very small steps that you know you can manage. Tell yourself that you can do it. Say, "Yes, I can."

Over time, Charlotte's internal dialogue became less like competition and more like reasonable negotiation. It took on a gentler but more honest tone and became even more effective.

That's a terrific tone to take. Don't be too harsh on yourself! And if this internal dialogue doesn't work the first time, then try it again. Reason eventually will prevail; I guarantee it.

You're All Too Human

The purpose of fine-tuning your internal dialogue is to transcend self-criticism and to become a reliable advocate for your effort. You need to accept that one little relapse does not justify retreat, and that gradual change is par for the course. There's no sense in beating yourself up because you still give into your chocolate cravings. If you were a daily chocoholic, you need to adjust your internal dialogue to acknowledge even a ramp down to a five times a week indulgence. Cutting out chocolate twice a week is a major accomplishment! You are entitled to take pride in that.

Your internal dialogue should reassure you that stress and failure are normal parts of life and shouldn't always have negative interpretations. As you gain more command over it, internal dialogue often can affect other aspects of your life that are related to your food issues, although they might seem distinct from them. This can be an extraordinary discovery.

Samantha was someone who figured this out. When we met, she would talk as much about money as she would about food. In fact, I think she cried and complained more about her finances! As she took the small weight-loss steps that soon grew into larger ones, the complaints about money diminished along with her extra weight.

I knew we were nearing the end of our time together when she told me that she was applying all of her weight-loss strategies to her relationship with money. She'd cut way down on her binge drinking for health reasons, but this also left her with far more disposable income. She figured out exactly how much less she was spending on food and bar bills every week, and she put that money into a savings account. After a few months, she was extremely happy about her growing nest egg, and felt much more in control about her weight, her money, and her life. I was incredibly proud of her savvy attitude and hard work!

But there is a flip side to Samantha's experience; sometimes your internal dialogue is hard to change because it protects you from dark emotions you aren't quite prepared to deal with. Those emotions lead to a great deal of sabotage. Negative body image is a common culprit.

Most women I've talked to have a certain degree of shame and/or loathing for their bodies when they are overweight. Yet once they slim down, these same women tell me that they feel uncomfortable in their new, sexier shape. Often, being overweight allows women to avoid unwanted male attention and to elude their own complicated and sometimes repressed feelings about sexuality. A great many conflicted feelings can be hidden by extra weight.

Carlotta is a good example. Born in Malta, she had stunning Mediterranean looks: golden honey skin; thick, wavy, dark-brown hair; huge, almond-shaped eyes; and a sweet and gleaming smile. Once she lost weight and followed a regular exercise regimen, she literally stopped traffic. People stared at her—the men leered wolfishly, and women gaped out of admiration and jealousy. It all made Carlotta very uncomfortable; she had no idea how to cope with being attractive to men or admired by anyone. She confessed to me that she wished she hadn't lost all that weight and wanted to gain it back. Her new life was too much to handle.

Fortunately, Carlotta didn't backslide; she came up with a terrific strategy instead. She worked with a therapist to confront her discomfort around sexuality. She gained a few pounds and felt much more comfortable in her own skin while maintaining a healthy, normal weight. Gradually, she could accept how she looked and how men reacted to her. Within a year, she was seeing a very nice guy who adored her and loved her body.

On the other hand, Sheila bounced in to see me one day, full of sass and smiles. "I am just so happy I did this!" she announced. "Now that I've lost all this weight, I've got all these guys after me. It's just one date after another. Can you believe it?!"

Yes, indeed I could.

The Saboteurs around You

When you are on track with a gradual, uncritical program of weight loss and the results are beginning to show, friends and family are going to comment. I'm hoping that you get plenty of nonjudgmental, encouraging feedback, but be prepared for comments that, however well-intentioned they might seem, make you feel uncomfortable, hurt, angry, or leave you questioning the value of your weight loss. Some people will make you very self-conscious as you try to take control.

Whether they know it or not, these people are saboteurs. It won't help you at all to leave them unnamed: you won't overcome the effects of their influence unless you see this negative feedback for what it is. Almost every successful client has told me about these challenges, many presented by people who were well intentioned and even (to their own mind) complimentary!

Why does it happen that other people can undermine a process that is personal (this is *your* waistline we're talking about, after all!), responsible, and validating? There's no simple answer, but consider one of the most obvious explanations first: fat literally is contagious.

In 2007, *The New England Journal of Medicine* published a report of the Framingham (Massachusetts) Heart Study, which analyzed a wealth of data collected over thirty-two years from 12,067 participants. The report's title, "The Spread of Obesity in a Large Social Network over 32 Years," says it all. A key finding of the study was that if a person has friends who are obese, his or her chances of also becoming obese are elevated by *57 percent*!

I believe this is an important case of data analysis bearing out the truth we see in front of our eyes every day. And that key finding should drive home a critical point: our attitudes toward food are communal, and we reinforce each other's eating habits. The common weight denominator of a group, whether it's a family network or social peers, affects all members.

Here's a perfect example of this concept in action. A couple of years ago I was in Cannes. I was in a restaurant, relishing my filet steak with salad and a glass of red wine. Idly, I was taking in the chatter of other diners until a couple, both severely overweight, captured my attention as they discussed the menu.

"Hmm, the baked chicken and veggies sounds delicious," said the wife.

"Sure does,' said the husband. "So does the grilled fish."

"Nice and healthy and fresh," she added.

"Yeah, we are on the Mediterranean, after all. We should eat local." They looked at each other and smiled lovingly.

Then silence.

The waiter came by. "Let's see. I'll have the fried fish and fries," said the wife as she handed him the menu, "with a large Coke."

"Yeah, same for me," said the husband.

Halfway through the meal, they each ordered another large Coke and more fries.

I left the restaurant saddened. I could only hope one of them would eventually find the strength to break this pattern of codependency. One of them could have deviated from the pattern by ordering the grilled chicken. But neither did.

Dealing with Friends and Sabotage

How often have you told a friend you're dieting, only to have him or her reply, "But you look fine just the way you are! Come on, why would you want to lose weight?"

I acknowledge that many of these comments come from a place of kindness, even love. But imagine: You've done some hard work. You've accepted that you want to change your lifestyle, and you're tackling your own inner saboteur and fear of change in an attempt to move forward. And then this: "What's the point? You're great as you are!"

Trust me, it won't sound like kindness. It will sound cruel. And often it is, even if the person doesn't mean to be.

A truly kind reaction is more like this: "OK, sounds like you have a plan. Let me know what I can do to keep you on track." Or perhaps, "I'm so happy for you. That's great. Do you have any tips for me? I could stand to lose a few pounds; can we can do this together?"

Now, to be fair, many unhelpful comments come *after* a new dieter has embarked on a lecture that emphasizes the virtue of their actions. If you have overweight friends, they're probably just as sensitive about their conditions as you are about yours. And they don't have to be paranoid to hear your recital about the dangers of sugar addiction and figure you're really talking about *them*.

Try not to be a diet bore. When you are in the initial stages of your weight-loss program, it's probably best not to challenge the standards of a group. Find a confidante with whom you can discuss your challenges, but be wary of falling into old role play. Maybe you've been the one in your social circle who raves about diets, who is sure that *this time* it's going to work. Announcements and lectures simply will perpetuate the standing story: you announce, and the group expects you to fail. When you do, they offer assurances and comfort, which is easy since they feel no pressure to confront their own problems with extra weight. It's easy to reinforce bad habits within a group; it's much harder to think for one's self.

Habits are, after all, very hard to break. Your group of friends may be appalled if you suggest eating anywhere but the local pizza restaurant where you always go—and where they know you'll have a hard time finding anything healthy to eat. Your attempts to lose weight may win admiration, until you question the weekend ritual of watching games, eating junk, and drinking beer. Some friends will feel hurt if they can't cook your favorite high-calorie meals for you anymore; they'll fear your rejection and may lash out with ridicule. Consciously or unconsciously, friends can become weight-loss enemies (not *your* enemies!) if you let them.

Of course, ignorance is often the culprit behind insensitivity. Many friends are conditioned to expressing affection by minimizing our problems. "OK, maybe you could lose a couple of pounds," one might say when you, after taking your measurements and doing research, know you could lose forty. This friend probably cares for you very much; he or she simply doesn't realize that it no longer helps for you to avoid the truth.

Best Solution: Be Direct

Any solution to these tricky problems probably won't sit well with Advice Askers and Victims, because a real solution requires taking control of the situation. In most cases, the best way to do that is to be straightforward.

Unwitting saboteurs can become supporters if you explain the situation calmly and objectively. This is a good time to present facts (but without a lecture). "I know you're trying to be supportive when you say I don't need to lose weight, but let's be honest here," you might say. "The reality is that I'm easily forty pounds overweight. I don't want to risk my health. I'm working on losing it."

In uncomplicated relationships, being direct can clear the air and quickly lead to firmer friendship and support. But even if friendship doesn't quickly track in a new, positive direction, the direct approach has a benefit of telling you a great deal about your friend.

Watch his or her reaction closely. You may sense that your friend is wrestling with the little demon, jealousy. Perhaps she's afraid you soon will be more attractive; maybe she's used to you being "the fat one" while she, the "cute one," often has felt secure at your expense! After you own up to your intention to lose weight, your friend might retort by questioning your conclusion: you're really not *that* fat, she might say. Then again, maybe she'll goad you into dining out or accepting quick snacks. These are attempts to reestablish the old terms of the friendship.

Your perceptions will help you to understand why your friend isn't supportive. Unfortunately, not every situation will have a happy ending. Some people are not able to adjust when their friends make a concentrated effort to change, and they never become comfortable with their friends' weight loss. There may be nothing else to this particular bond; in these cases, you'll do best to move on and find new friendships where you're accepted as a Decision Maker.

But in many cases, you can help the friendship shift by being clear about your intentions and allowing others to get used to the new you gradually. Whether the friends are fat or thin, you'll send a warm message by seeking them out and appreciating them as you always have, even as you are changing and shedding weight. Remember that many people will fear that you no longer have use for them once you succeed; you can calm those fears by showing that you're still you, no matter how many pounds you're carrying or losing.

Dealing with Saboteurs during a Meal

Shared mealtimes are tricky. The menu may be delicious, tempting, and high in calories. You'll hear things like "Just try a little bit" or "A slice of cake won't put back all the weight you've lost" or even "You know, too much dieting can lead to eating disorders."

True, there's no cake in the world that is so caloric that it will replace a few weeks of lost weight in a single slice. But remember that the initial stages of your weight loss will be difficult; as I described in chapter two, you'll be in sugar detox for several weeks. Staying far away from sugar is critical: patter about "just a little bit" and eating disorders is undermining behavior. However innocent it is meant to be, it's anything but.

By now our society realizes that telling a friend in Alcoholics Anonymous to "have just one little drink" would be stupid and cruel. I'm hopeful that one day soon, sugar detoxers will receive more consideration, too. But until then, you may well have to fight for respect and commit to nipping undermining behavior in the bud.

Excuses, Excuses

Look, I'm as uncomfortable with making excuses as the next person. But when food peer pressure catches you flat-footed, I think a little dissembling is a much lesser evil than undoing a lot of good work. In fact, an adept excuse is a lesser art form of sorts, and recovering alcoholics, to name one group, have been refining their lines for years.

Sometimes a little song and dance is necessary to help us wiggle through socially awkward moments. As you attempt to maintain your weight-loss program, you'll sometimes have to justify what you are (or are not) putting in your mouth. You should be ready with some responses that will not embarrass or humiliate anyone, or leave people skeptical and inquisitive.

Excuses don't have to hurt anybody's feelings; they may well *prevent* feelings being hurt. And if that excuse leaves you in control over what's on your plate and in your glass, it's useful.

Here are a few means to handle saboteurs and well-meaning but non-comprehending hosts:

* I'll have an appetizer while you get your main course. I love the appetizers here.

* I had such a big lunch today; I'd rather stay light tonight.

* I really came more for the company than the food.

* Got a new client interview tomorrow and quite lost my appetite.
* Tomorrow I have a family lunch with my mom's specials.

If you play it smart and don't announce that you're out to lose weight, many of these statements can protect you without any flap being raised. Most people don't need to know what you're up to, after all. These excuses should act as deflections; the message should be a polite, but firm, request that others mind their own business.

Reverse the Sabotage

Sometimes, you can go on the offensive against the saboteurs. And have fun with it!

Say to your friend, "I need to park at the far end of the lot so I can get some extra walking in today. Do you mind walking with me?" How many people will say, "I do mind. Drop me at the door and do your walking yourself"? Chances are they'll walk with you and discover that taking a few extra steps really isn't so hard. You may even help them start walking on a healthier path, too.

Getting informed is often the best preparation. Since most people really don't know much about healthy food, citing a report or the advice of a professional will often keep you on safe ground. Make your doctor into the ultimate authority: "That looks delicious. Too bad the doctor just ordered me to reduce blood sugar and cholesterol." Doctors don't always have the last word, but this is one time when you can use their authority for protection.

Coworkers and Sabotage

The workplace can be a challenge to any diet; I often have clients who lapse because they don't want to spoil the camaraderie of a team. It's especially tough if you have coworkers who like to eat and bring in food for everyone. Casual Friday often kicks off with a spread of tempting doughnuts and muffins around breakfast; maybe it's your turn to buy them. A cake will come out for the office birthday party: "My wife made this!" It's all hard to resist, especially if it's your boss you don't want to offend!

Fortunately, you can always use the excuse that you've got work to do (one client even faked phone conversations when a coworker walked around with the doughnuts). But when you become the subject of water cooler chitchat, do your best to avoid the Big Announcement or bragging. If someone declares that you now look terrific and wants to know how it was done, be modest. Think about your weight loss as you would a sudden spike in income; you wouldn't gloat to your colleagues about the raise you just received, would you? Set a polite but careful tone at work, and avoid food discussions unless someone seeks you out for some serious conversation or advice.

When and if it comes time to address the subject of all the high-calorie snacks in the workroom, assume that you aren't going to score many points if you start throwing your lost weight around. Lobbying for the removal of pastries from coffee breaks by pointing out all the extra pounds everyone else is carrying will *not* be endearing, nor will it encourage anyone else to take your side.

But when it's your turn to bring in snacks, you can introduce seasonal fruits (with a little chocolate yogurt for dipping) without a lot of fanfare. Put some thought into your choices and make them memorable. If you're an Advice Asker, you might get the whole office involved by asking your coworkers to recommend healthier food alternatives; these suggestions could be posted somewhere, and you could all work together to try these healthier foods.

Other changes can be introduced quietly, such as swapping out the half-and-half for whole milk and then, if no one complains, a reduced-fat milk for coffee and tea. If there are candies or jellybeans for the taking, try placing a dish of raw almonds next to those items. If your replacements are popular, then push for other healthy choices. You won't know what's possible unless you try.

Family

I've saved the toughest for last. Weight issues tend to run in families, due to shared culture, cuisine, and holiday gatherings—in short, everything that makes a family a family. Food is present in our memories, traditions, and closest bonds. It's been a vehicle for parents (and Italian grandmothers!) to express love for their children. Food is often the means of welcoming friends and newcomers by marriage.

One of my clients told me a family legend about his grandfather Marvin. When he was courting his wife, the time came for Marvin to meet her grandmother. The traditional Jewish occasion for such a meeting is Shabbos dinner of cholent, a slow-baked dish made with beef, barley, and beans. It's delicious, but like a lot of traditional Eastern European Jewish cooking, very heavy. Marvin was warned if he wanted to get married, he sure better like Grandma's cholent.

The big day came. Marvin skipped breakfast and lunch, and sat down to a big bowl of cholent. He ate it all, praised it, and asked for more. Grandma brought a second bowl; he ate, praised, and asked for more. But the cholent got him in the end; though he struggled manfully, he could only get halfway through that third bowl.

Grandma stared at him and said, "What, you didn't like it?"

Poor Marvin! I can only hope he wasn't trying to lose weight then. But his story illustrates why diets can be so hard to maintain during family gatherings. A stuffed son (or son-in-law) is a loved son. You may be afraid that your new diet plans will be perceived as rejection by the people you most care about. I sympathize; when I needed to lose weight at ten, I surely didn't want my Italian grandmother to think I was rejecting her food. Who could refuse such delicious fare? I may have been overweight, but I certainly wasn't crazy.

Where do you think the concept of "comfort food" originated? Right in family kitchens. Maybe you have weakness for fried chicken and buttery mashed potatoes because those rich smells and hearty tastes bring you right back to childhood. But be aware that those good feelings invoked by the memories *are not about the food itself.* They are emotions born from the feelings of security and belonging that come with communal family eating.

Why is that an important distinction? Because it will help you to realize that you don't have to "reject" the family food. You can still praise it all and give a particularly loud shout-out to the healthier dishes. And I know that if I could lose weight by eating a little less of what my *nonna* put in front of me when I was a kid, you can rein in your appetite just enough at family gatherings to sustain your weekly balance of food and exercise.

At home, too, you should avoid open discussion of your plans. Family dynamics are always complicated, and it's harder to control other members' responses if you hit them over the head with your intention to eat less. Studies have shown that kids of overweight parents have an 80 percent chance of becoming overweight themselves. Meanwhile, if the parents believe that their extra weight is normal, they don't perceive their kids as being too heavy, even if their health is at risk. This should help you understand why some family members are puzzled by or unsupportive of your weight loss. Even if they, too, are heavy, they may well have no understanding of why you would want to lose weight.

So you need to have a game plan for family dinners, one that is realistic about your chance—and your desire—of breaking free of old trends. Keep your expectations reasonable: you aren't going to reform your entire clan. You just need to make sure that *you*—not sabotaging family members—are in control of what you eat.

The simplest approach is to not change at all. If your family gathers for Sunday dinner, make Sunday your free day and eat what you want. You don't break ranks, you'll enjoy what you eat, and you can spend the rest of the week keeping up your new eating schedule.

But if this isn't convenient, or if you sit down with family more often, there are other options. Discreetly eat less of the foods you know you should avoid and more of the ones you should be eating. Put more protein, which is sugar free (fish, meat, poultry, and so on) on your plate so you can have smaller portions of the more calorie-dense items (rice, breads, pasta, fried food). If you do this without calling attention to yourself, without refusing to eat a lovingly prepared family favorite because "it's not allowed," chances are nobody will really notice the size of your portion.

If you're uncomfortable with these methods, or if you think others in your family are open to changing old habits, by all means try honesty. Plenty of my clients came from families that gradually changed their eating habits as a show of support. Not all families are resistant to changes (just as not all friends are). If you're hopeful, put your intentions on the table, so to speak.

Your Spouse or Partner

There's not much good in hiding here. Any serious change a person undertakes will affect his or her spouse, for good or ill or perhaps both. Whether your partner realizes it or not, your attempts to lose weight could aggravate all sorts of insecurities.

Paula worked as a cleaning lady and had a terrible time with her husband, Mark, when she started losing weight. He was constantly belittling her and undermining everything she tried (her revamped recipes, her household junk-food purge, her exercising). The more she lost, the more Mark put her down. Their home life became bitter.

Finally (this was Paula's Decision Maker taking over), she confronted Mark about his bad attitude. To her amazement, he burst into tears. It turned out Mark feared that losing weight would make Paula beautiful again, and she'd leave him for someone else.

Paula replied, "But, honey, I'm not just doing this for me. I am doing this for *you*, to be more attractive to you, not so I can find another man!"

Paula and Mark had been married for many years, and had gotten into a bit of a rut. They'd stopped talking about their intimate hopes and fears, and wound up completely misunderstanding each other. It was easy for Mark to hallucinate about Paula's goals.

I don't believe you can tiptoe around the person you live with. Paula did the right thing by calling Mark to account. Once he realized that her goal was not to throw him over, he did an about-face and became very supportive. As for Paula, her weight loss gave her more energy, and she easily worked longer hours and brought in more money. Her clients noticed her new shape and lifestyle and asked what she was eating. Then they asked her to shop for them and cook a few meals! Paula's weight loss helped her to move up from simple cleaning services to professional housekeeping, all while reviving some spark in her marriage. Weight loss can pay off in a lot of different ways.

Of course, plenty of spouses jump right on board with weight loss; I've consulted with many husbands who wanted to know how they could best support their wives. I always remind these men that weight loss is a long process, with good and bad days, so interested neutrality is always a good position to take. By asking "How's the weight loss going?" or "Tell me about your program" or "Is there anything you'd like me to do?" they show their wives that they're present, without being critical or judgmental, and willing to provide loving conversation and emotional support.

I had a good laugh with one hubby once when he told me he didn't like to go to the supermarket with his wife anymore. She'd learned so much about nutrition and healthy eating that she couldn't stop criticizing what was in everyone else's carts. I told him she was just going through a phase and she'd get over it in a few weeks, which she did. And he learned a lot about nutritious choices, too, so he could do their food shopping on his own.

Your Children

It's important for families to eat together as often as possible; this is the foundation of good eating habits. I know how hard this can be if you have several children of varying ages, but once family mealtime is established, you can start making small, subtle changes that I doubt your kids will even notice. You can stop serving juice at dinner and replace it with flavored water. You can make your own vinaigrette instead of using creamy salad dressing. You can buy takeaway or frozen dinners that are the least processed and the most nutritious once you've raised your nutritional IQ and become savvy about reading labels. Or, instead of pizza night, you can have a chicken and roasted potatoes night. As long as you make it fun and delicious and not about deprivation, your kids will embrace the new approach.

Here's a suggestion that works well: ask your kids, one at a time, to write down what they like to eat most. Tell them they can write whatever they want. They very well may surprise you.

Here is a sample list written by Jack, who is ten and the son of a client:

* The white meat with crust (When asked to specify, he said he meant chicken and turkey with roasted skin still on.)

* Potatoes

* Vegetables mashed all together

* Pineapple

* All fruit with chocolate sauce (He meant dipping sauce.)
* Mummy's pizza
* Fried fish (He meant calamari.)
* Corn with butter
* Lollies

The reaction from his mother was interesting: "Oh my! I never buy pineapple but our neighbor does. He told me he prefers roasted potatoes with cheese to fried chips, which I would give him because I thought all kids liked chips better than roasted potatoes. On pizza night I always order one pizza for him and another for myself; I had no idea he wanted mine." (It turned out the pizzas had very similar caloric values.) "And I would have never imagined he would put corn on his list. "

I was particularly curious about the "vegetables mashed all together," so I asked Jack about it. He explained that he would love to have all his vegetables in one bowl and mashed because "it would taste much better." I agreed! I tried my own version: broccoli, carrots, potatoes, and cauliflower all mashed together. It was delicious. And now Jack's mum makes her own variation for him all the time.

If you're a parent, you've had to embrace decision making and control to some extent; once you're losing weight you'll want to tap into that authority. Children learn what "normal" is from their parents, so you have great power to define healthy eating as an everyday activity for everyone in your family. You might have a struggle shifting your kids' consciousness away from old favorites—all those sugared cereals and Happy Meals are marketed right at them—and indeed, you might feel you're depriving them of happiness. But you must remember that fast-food advertisements, filled with smiles and healthy faces, don't show the realty of junk-food addiction. Marketing has nothing to do with the truth. Its sole function is to persuade; often it's to persuade you to buy something you don't really need or want. Ask yourself if what the subliminal messages are selling is a must-have. Don't fall for the hype.

With a little hard work and determination, your entire family can start eating better. And you'll be instilling habits that can last a lifetime.

But again, gently does it! It is vital that you don't become obsessive nag. Research into the epidemic of eating disorders in young women and men shows that many come from families where one parent, almost always the mother, is constantly dieting or talking about it. In one study, 45 percent of girls said that their mothers encouraged them to diet. This unhealthy preoccupation with weight, dieting, and eating the "right" foods can set the stage for eating disorders such as anorexia, bulimia, binge eating, and severe obesity.

Kids are blessed with super-charged metabolism, and most love to be active. There's no need for obsession. Make sure they're exercising, and encourage them to eat plenty of the food you now know is good for them. Try to avoid saying that cakes and candy are rewards for being good. Teach them to embrace a love of healthy food; with that love, they can then gain control of their own relationships with food in adulthood.

Back to You

I don't think I've ever counseled a person who was a virgin dieter. By the time they found me, my clients either had attempted many diets or watched friends and family struggle with weight loss. Many of them were very knowledgeable about exercise, calorie counts, and why sugar is bad for them. They had used programs with prepared meals. They had been supported and encouraged by diet buddies. And despite all that support and knowledge, nothing had worked for them in the long run. Many had become depressed, discouraged, and disparaging.

The key to lasting success is self-support. Hopefully, your peers and family will provide plenty of encouragement, but if you control your internal dialogue—keeping it positive no matter what happens—you can lose your weight whether you have external support or not. When you are positive about you, you *will* effect change in your environment. The saboteurs can be neutralized. You can even swing them over to your side.

The essential cheerleader is the one you see in the mirror. Always be your own advocate.

Summary

- *Once you have begun to lose weight or have reached your goal weight, you might have to work against weight-loss sabotage.*

- *Sabotage can come from many sources, including friends, family, coworkers, the media, and yourself.*

- *It's easy to become frightened by the changes in your body when you begin to lose weight; you will need to deal with the internal issues that caused you to become overweight in the first place such as anxiety, insecurity, lack of self-confidence, and a desire to please others.*

- *Being prepared to respond wisely when placed in situations where individuals encourage you to make unwise food decisions will help you prevent weight-loss sabotage.*

- *Avoid the sabotage of your weight-loss success by not making a big deal of your changed eating habits and gradually getting friends and family used to your new body.*

- *Advocate for your children by instilling good eating habits in them at an early age. Make good health a family affair.*

- *Resist sabotage in the form of media images.*

Chapter Eight

EMOTIONAL EATING

F ood is essential to all living creatures. Without adequate nutrition, we die. For humans, food is central to celebration, family, and special events of all kinds. Food and its preparation are one of the few things all cultures value.

So how did things get so out of balance? Why do so many of us not only eat to live but also live to eat? Why do so many people eat when they aren't hungry, compelled by an irrational need to fill themselves with food? Why is the relationship between food and emotions so powerful?

These are all enormous questions that reach beyond the scope of any single book. But we're going to take a quick look at factors that influence emotional eating so that you can be on the alert in those quiet hours, when your emotions come through loud and clear. Remember, unhealthy weight gain is rarely due to ignorance alone. In almost every case there is a strong emotional component to the problem. This chapter will provide you with some tools to break the habit of emotional eating.

The Roots of Emotional Eating

Emotional eating is initiated by a hunger for feelings, not nutrients. Sometimes, we eat to suppress unpleasant emotions such as anger, depression, loneliness, grief, and anxiety.

We *feel* emotional hunger in between the breast and the bellybutton. Bad emotional experiences arrive like a punch "in the pit of the stomach." We describe anxiety as "butterflies in the stomach"; we get stomachaches and stomach ulcers from stress. Emotions can manifest as a huge hole in our middle that needs filling, much as real hunger does.

For most of us, our emotional eating has its origins in early childhood, when adults lovingly rewarded or comforted us with food. If you scraped your knee, your mother cleaned it up and then handed you a cookie. When you were a good girl or boy, you got a cookie. When the adults around you felt guilty, they handed you a cookie (or bought you a new car, but one emotional complication per book!). Pretty soon, comfort and food were linked together, a cause and effect.

My father was always traveling on business. I often became upset when he left. He saw my feelings but felt he could do little to assuage them. Except drop a big box of chocolates in my lap whenever he left on a trip.

In my mind, insecurity, love, self-comfort, and feeling deserted all merged into one giant chocolate. As I grew older, chocolate's power to soothe me only deepened.

I'm sorry to tell all the hardworking parents this, but giving your kids bananas or string beans as an emotional sop probably won't work. Comfort foods almost exclusively are those items that are high in sugar, carbs, and fat. Look back to chapter two for the explanation: the sweet taste of sugar stimulates the production of serotonin, your body's natural feel-good chemical. Fat, meanwhile, stimulates endorphin production. Fat and sugar: chocolate, anyone?

In a downer situation, you crave an emotional lift. A sugary, fatty food affects the brain the same way that opiates do; it provides a comparable lift. Not only that, but sugar acts directly on the brain to inhibit the effect of leptin, a natural hormone in our bodies. This causes us to never feel full.

Brain chemistry helps explains why we don't turn to celery sticks as a tonic. Celery just doesn't have what it takes. So we turn to mac and cheese, mashed potatoes, cheese curls, chocolate, cakes, cookies, and other sugary and salty snacks. And of course, these foods often are what parents give their kids for treats, thereby creating a vicious cycle.

Of course, there are plenty of occasions when the pairing of food and emotion is a wonderful thing that provides a foundation of many wonderful memories. But you, in becoming a savvy, more alert eater, will be able to differentiate between cherished moments and juvenile coping mechanisms that have extended into adulthood. Wedding cake on your Big Day is one thing; secret midnight binges of pizza and potato chips is quite another.

Overeating Because You're Stressed and/or Unhappy

Getting through life isn't easy; stress is a natural byproduct of life. It's also one of the major causes of overeating.

Some people, rather than eating, take pills to deal with stress. This hasn't erased the problem of emotional eating; it's simply created a whole new population of medicated worriers. Antidepressants can work, of course; when prescribed properly for those who truly need them, Prozac, Xanax, and other drugs have been very useful. But some people who rely on antidepressants become so "relaxed" that they no longer feel like exercising, which opens them up to some familiar problems.

We could debate endlessly whether these medications are overprescribed. But what can't be ignored is that these are powerful substances that have created some unpleasant side effects—including, most notably, weight gain and overall slowdown of the metabolism. This can lead to decreased energy, reduced will to exercise, and sleep pattern change. Each of these changes can have a severe effect on any weight-loss plan.

Alexa was someone who found this out. She had been taking psychiatric medications for nearly twenty years when she came to me. She told me she really wanted to work out regularly to augment her weight-loss plans, but whenever she tried she just didn't have the energy. She felt she didn't need the drugs anymore—she was newly secure in her job, and her anxiety had diminished considerably.

I told her to run all of this past her doctor who, if he agreed, would help her through the cessation process. (You must *never* try to wean yourself off these medications without medical guidance.) As soon as the drug was out of her system, she was amazed by how much energy she had. She's now a regular in the gym, has slimmed down, and is brimming with health and vitality.

I'll disclose my own point of view here: I believe that the sedation of anxiety in an otherwise mentally healthy person is repression, not treatment. It's not getting to the root cause of the anxiety; it's only treating the symptom, and not treating it well.

But one way or the other, you must deal with anxiety and understand the role it's playing in your life. Ignore it, and you'll eventually explode. The compounding stress of anxiety repression may very well lead to some form of stress-related illness.

Of course, many suppress anxiety simply by eating it. A cookie, a thick slab of bread, a chocolate bar: these things may neutralize unhealthy anxiety momentarily, but they never uproot it.

Try to differentiate between healthy, normal worrying and debilitating anxiety. There is a difference. A life with no worries at all wouldn't be terribly interesting, and some worries spring from our desire to solve problems, which certainly is a healthy impulse. Look out for anxieties that serve no purpose, which sap you of energy and contribute nothing positive at all.

Sometimes, having a good, long, focusing think about anxiety helps pinpoint its triggers. Does your family cause you anxiety? Are you concerned about your relationship with your spouse or a friend? Are you worried about your finances? Is your career where you want it to be? Do you have a loved one dealing with illness?

As you are thinking about the causes of your anxiety, start to look at possible solutions to these problems. If you cannot think of solutions right away, that's OK. At least you'll be conscious of your worry, and hopefully, it won't masquerade as hunger; this is the unconscious beginning of an emotional eating habit.

Dangers in the Night

Another major stress factor is lack of sleep. Worry, shift work, and staying up late in an attempt to squeeze more hours into your day can all lead to deprivation.

More and more research shows that lack of sleep is directly linked to anxiety and weight gain. When you don't get your usual seven to eight hours of sleep each night, your body chemistry and metabolism are thrown off. In particular, the hormones ghrelin and leptin, which play a big role in regulating your appetite, get out of balance. Ghrelin tells you you're hungry and should eat, while leptin monitors your overall body fat and curbs your appetite. When you don't get enough sleep, even for just a couple of days, your body produces *more* ghrelin and *less* leptin. You begin to crave high-calorie carbohydrates. Overall, your metabolism slows when you don't sleep enough. It's a situation ideal for gaining weight.

Nervous Energy and Boredom

Some people have a lot of nervous energy that manifests as an oral fixation. They need to be doing something with their mouths almost every minute of the day. Many need weight-loss help because what they do most often with their mouths is eat. I can spot this nervous energy in an instant. It makes people fidgety, so they smoke, chew their nails, and talk constantly. And eat.

Helping these people find achievable ways to lose weight is fairly straightforward. They're comforted or relaxed by moving their mouths; they may or may not notice the taste of the food. We talk about ways to make better food choices that still allow them to chew a lot. It generally helps to substitute high-caloric snack food with sugarless gums, or even straws in a bottle of water or toothpicks. This cuts out a lot of excess calories but keep their oral fixations satisfied.

How many times have you found yourself in the kitchen, scouring the shelves for something tasty because you just felt like having something to do? I am absolutely guilty of this! I can catch myself now, give myself a little shake, and leave the kitchen in pursuit of something more interesting. Well, most of the time.

Boredom, perhaps the flip side of stress, also is an emotional condition conducive to weight gain. We eat to have something to do while waiting to pick up the kids, or to kill time before the movie starts, or to distract ourselves from a tedious task. If you have a nibble every time you have a little lull during your day, you can end up taking in a lot more calories than you realize, and many more than you need.

Simply being aware that you're prone to eating out of boredom is the first step in cutting back. I think the best solution would be to pick a hobby, and fast, but if you're still inclined to eat, take a cue from chapter one and substitute; if you're going to graze to pass the time, graze in a healthy pasture!

Overeating Because You Want to Please

Many people have told me that one of the reasons they could not change their lifestyle and their eating habits was because of their families. They said under no circumstances would their mother/grandmother/sister/lover/partner accept that they were changing their eating and nutrition habits.

This is a classic blind spot. It's unbelievable how stubborn all those mothers and spouses are! Victims the world over rely on these kitchen autocrats to keep them helpless against weight gain.

Consider that you might be stuck because of what you assume another person will do or not do. Here are a few examples of clients who stopped guessing about what *might happen* and overcame the family pressure:

"I put a lot less food on my plate, and she didn't even notice!" Suzanna reported after a Sunday family lunch at her mum's. "I can't believe it! I spent all these years eating a ton of food because I thought that's what she wanted. I'm just shocked. It was all in my head!"

"I told my sister my blood sugar was really high and I had to be very careful about what I was eating," Nancy said. "And she just asked me what I wanted her to cook for my next visit."

"I finally got the courage to tell my mom I was trying to lose weight," Abby said. "And she told me she really wanted to lose weight, too, and asked if we could do this together. Diana, my mum wants to come, too, so we can support each other. We're going to encourage each other and learn a lot more about how to eat. My only regret is that I didn't bring this up sooner, because we would be much further along with our weight loss!"

Victims, take note of these stories. In each one, there was an intractable person who had control over the food supply. Two assumptions there: intractability and control. *And they both were figments of the victim's imagination!*

You do not have to be a victim of your assumptions. Just consider the possibility that your loved one is *not* the weight-loss enemy you suspect him or her to be. Advice Askers, take this advice: decide to make a change.

We spend a great deal of time with our families, and over the years, walls of misperception and missed signals become imposing. Eventually, we don't react to our relatives so much out of what we know but what we *think* we know. The reality of your relative's mindset might be very different from what you've imagined. Maybe your mother desperately wants you to bring up the topic of food and cooking and overeating because she doesn't know how to do it herself. Maybe her menu is a habit she's sick of, but she thinks it's what you want. Maybe she thinks she's pleasing *you* by making those meatballs you now know are too caloric. The question is, have you ever sat down with your loved ones and told them what you want?

We make half-baked assumptions all the time, especially when it comes to family. You don't know what loved ones really think or feel unless you ask them. If you can find a gentle way of bringing up what's important to you, you may be pleasantly surprised by the response you get.

After all, most family members want what's best for you. It's healthier for both your mind and your waistline to communicate openly with the people in your life. Communicating effectively may take practice, but you can do it. "No," you may be thinking, "I can't tell my mother what I really need." To this I would say, "Yes, you can."

The Overeating Habit

Joanie was sitting in a comfortable chair, telling me about her older sister, who as a child and teenager was strong and muscled but always a bit on the chunky side. One night, when they were teens, they went to a Mexican restaurant with their parents and ate a delicious dinner of *chilies rellenos* and refried beans and a big container of chips and salsa. Joanie didn't overdo it, but she was stuffed after such a rich and filling meal.

Half an hour later, they were home, watching TV. Joanie went to the bathroom and returned to find her sister eating a plate of hard-boiled eggs.

"That's why I remember it," Joanie told me with a wry smile. "Because I was so incredibly full and I couldn't believe my sister didn't feel the same. I asked her how she could be hungry, because I couldn't believe she really was."

I smiled back. "She wasn't really hungry," I explained. "It's not about fullness. It was a *habit*."

"What do you mean?" Joanie asked.

"I'll bet that for her, back then, whether she was going to school, staying home, or having a Mexican meal with her family, she was used to coming back home and going to the refrigerator. She probably had no idea she even did it."

Coming home and going to the kitchen for a snack is an extremely common habit. It may have started when you were a kid and came home starving from school. As an adult, you may be hungry and stressed after a long day at work, and you need something to tide you over until dinner.

Many people also eat late at night or after midnight out of habit. These people feel that they can't go to sleep without a something on their stomach. How often have you felt like eating something right before you go to bed, such as a piece toast, cheese, or a cookie? You may feel that you can never break your late-night eating habit. But guess what?

You can. Little by little, with some conscious thought and better planning, you can do it.

How to Fix Emotional Eating

Since reading chapter seven, I hope you've been working hard to shape your internal dialogue into a positive force of reassurance and insight. If you have, you can use that refurbished ID to tackle the root causes of your emotional eating and provide you with solutions.

When the next "reach-for-the-lifeline-in-the-fridge" moment occurs, give pause. Take a moment to acknowledge that yes, you are feeling pretty lousy today. Then take a deep breath and say, "So OK, I feel terrible today. And I know if I have that big bowl of ice cream I will feel even worse." Take another minute. Really let that observation sink in.

Maybe you'll stop short of grabbing a teaspoon, pulling out the carton, and digging in. Maybe you won't stop. But either way, you take ownership of the situation. If you ate the ice cream, it's because you chose to do it. You didn't mindlessly polish off the carton, and that's the key change: emotional eating, by its nature, is usually mindless activity; it's a gut-centered action. Try moving the action back into your head in that crucial moment.

Keep practicing. Build up a story until it's a mantra: "I am not going to eat that snack. I can be strong enough not to, and if I really need it, I will just have a bit. I really need to feel the satisfaction of saying no to a snack." And remember that the physical urge lasts for just fifteen minutes. That's it. All you need to do is to distract yourself for fifteen minutes, nine hundred seconds, a quarter of an hour. Whatever expression of time seems shortest to you, employ it.

The substitution rule can work well here, too, but I don't mean substituting one food for another. This time you'll swap activities, eating for something else that's pleasurable. Be honest about this. It may feel virtuous to work on your taxes instead of snacking, but if that's really no pleasure, it isn't likely to keep you clear of the ice cream container!

Probably you'll do better if you pick another activity that feels indulgent. Give yourself another treat. Read a book (trashy novels count), watch a movie, browse the Web, play with the dog, have sex, exercise, do yoga, work on a hobby, sing karaoke, or call a friend who sympathizes—whatever works for you.

Some people won't succeed if the focus remains on their desires; they need to look outside of themselves. In this situation, nothing works better than getting involved and keeping busy. So volunteer for a cause that's important to you, spend more time with your family, or take a class. Many people help themselves by helping others. If they're active and engaged, they're less likely to feel the need to soothe their feelings with ice cream or other low-quality foods.

Since this restless eating really isn't about hunger, I think it makes the most sense to steer clear of food. But if you absolutely must have something to eat *right now,* remember the substitution method from chapter one, and take the less desirable option, your second-favorite food.

I love milk chocolate the most, so I buy dark chocolate instead. A small amount satisfies my chocolate craving without triggering the childhood memories and overindulgence that milk chocolate would. One of my clients buys her least-favorite flavor of ice cream for the same reason.

Finding alternatives to emotional eating is an A-to-Z process like any other part of my weight-loss plan. In addition, keep in mind that the kind of eater you are will determine how you deal with your emotional eating.

If you're a Decision Maker, you will read this section, put the book down, and immediately come up with alternative activities to combat your emotional eating. You will schedule a regular power walking routine and exchange your chocolate chip cookies for fruit salad with a swirl of vanilla custard instead. Go for it! Just don't get so gung-ho that you forget all the rest of your obligations. Remember to start slow rather than leaping into a new routine without thinking it through.

If you're an Advice Asker you will eagerly read all the suggestions in this chapter, and then spend so much time wondering which one is for you that you may not follow any of them. Your challenge will be to pick one or two suggestions in this chapter, try them, and stick with the best.

If you're a Victim, you might head all the way back to the scene of the crime, so to speak, and feel bitter about the person who helped your anxiety take root so many years ago. You'll figure that *this person* is the one who needs help, not you. I can only point out that this is your emotional eating we're talking about, and your weight gain, which can expand your waistline and no one else's. Whoever helped create your troubles has done enough: Do you want this person to do more by keeping you at an unhealthy weight? Try to separate the problem of the moment (emotional medication with food) from deeper ones.

A True Story

I was a Nutella addict. I'd eat it right out of the jar with great satisfaction and delight. As I mentioned in chapter five, I actually tried the Nutella diet for a while, but even after my body delivered positive proof that this was a lousy idea, I kept binging on the stuff. I couldn't stop eating this sugary food even after I'd resumed an otherwise normal diet. My weight started creeping up.

Now I understand the physical component to my problem, and you probably can spot it too: almost certainly I was a sugar addict. But at the time, I concentrated on my state of mind. When at last I got fed up, I remember saying, "What can I do? *Why* am I doing this? Oh, I know, because it makes me happy. But does it really? No, the sugar fix is pleasurable, but the consequences, I hate them. Well, what other things make me happy? Let me see...well, shopping does!"

This, of course, is not what you'd advise your own daughter to do, but I was young, impulsive, and desperate to change my eating habits. I carefully placed my credit card in my wallet, one that luckily didn't have a huge credit limit on it, and set out for one of the best shopping experiences of my young life. It lasted an entire, blissful day. I maxed out the credit card and went home with my fabulous new shoes, handbags, perfume, and dresses. I spent two or three thousand dollars, which was a huge amount of money for me at the time. But I remember thinking, *Wow, I didn't spend one second thinking about food or Nutella or anything else that I'd used to fill myself up.* I'd succeeded in checking my impulse to eat bad food!

I'm sure you're wondering what I did when the bill came. Well, I tapped into my savings and paid it off. My irresponsibility did have a few limits.

But rather than start another negative ID, I sat and had another big think. Obviously, a shopping spree like that was a one-off; I knew I'd be working hard for a long time to replenish my now-empty savings account. *OK,* I thought.

I've learned it's possible to stop eating out of boredom. But I have to find other (cheaper!) ways of getting distracted. What are the other things that I can do to make me—not anyone else—filled up with happiness?

It was winter, the perfect time to draw a nice, hot, steamy bath with lots of exotic oils and soak. I had the oils already (thanks to the shopping spree). This indulgence wouldn't cost me an extra cent. So off I went.

That hour-long bath was especially blissful because afterward I went right to sleep. Like so many people, I felt keen food cravings at night and did most of my emotional eating after dark. The next morning I realized that with this lovely bath, I had replaced my bad habit of eating; there was nothing else—even binging on Nutella—that made me happier.

You can use this very same technique. Ask yourself, *When am I most likely to be an emotional eater?* Is it all day long, or are there certain times, like after work or close to bedtime? Are there specific triggers (calls from your family, problems at work, your boyfriend's or husband's moods)? Once you identify the trigger situations, you'll be able to move on to dealing with them. You will begin to experience an exhilarating feeling of control: control over your own body and your own mind.

Always Use Small Steps

Let's think back to my shopping spree. It had two big problems: it was unsustainable (unless I wanted to destroy my credit rating), and it was a big, outsized gesture. These rarely work. My program, by design, focuses on making a series of very small, subtle changes rather than one big one, which usually fails.

When most people start a "diet," all they think about is changing what they eat, whether the plan is restrictive enough, and if they can stick to it. They're not thinking about changing the *how*, the *why*, and the *when* of eating, which are all as important as *what* you eat.

Focusing on how, why, and when will help you pinpoint the emotional eating triggers. Without these efforts, you can learn everything about food, exercise, and calorie counts and fail anyway, because you are still the same person, whether you're dieting or not. The "just do it!" technique is fruitless when people continue to do everything else as they always have. The emotions and habits are not understood, and eventually, they overcome any superficial attempt to eat better.

But if you commit to making subtle, gradual changes in your routines and emotional reactions, weight loss will be much less of a struggle.

One of my best friends has been a smoker for years; her habit drives me crazy. It drives lots of other people who love her crazy, and they have no compunction about telling her just how bad smoking is for her. Is she deaf to these entreaties? Of course not! Does she want to quit? Of course she does! But *how* is she going to quit...*how* is she going to find a stop-smoking strategy that will really work...*how* will she stay off cigarettes for good once she does quit? Those were the all-important questions that none of her friends ever seemed to have answers for.

I finally got so fed up that I started applying my weight-loss strategies to her smoking addiction. I told her she was on a journey from A (smoking a pack a day) to Z (her not needing to smoke ever again). We worked on finding alternatives to lighting up, which she did mainly to quell her nervous energy. Has she quit yet? No, but she drastically reduced her smoking, from a pack of thirty to twelve and, presently, an average of just five cigarettes a day, with a few extra on the stressful days.

Am I still nagging her about smoking? No! I'm very proud of her for cutting down so much over time. I'd say she is somewhere around M in the A-to-Z process, and I have every faith that she's on track to quit soon.

So let's use this very same idea with overeating. Perhaps you have many people telling you how bad it is to be overweight. It's annoying—not only because it's rude of them, but also because *you already know this*! You know all about it (especially if you've been reading this book in sequence)!

But how many of these know-it-alls actually tell you *how* to stop the overeating and make the first step?

That's why my *how* always begins small. Little changes make a big difference. Some of these changes are within your diet. Some concern your meal plans and controlling your blood sugar. Some will make you aware of your emotional triggers. Truly effective and lasting weight loss is a project with many moving parts; you must be willing to give yourself sufficient time to master them all.

Use the Five-Times Method

The reinforcement of repetitive action is a phenomenon well-known to psychologists and many other professionals who try to exploit it. You can make it work for your weight loss, too, with what I call the Five-Times Method.

Dr. Rachel Holt, a neuro-linguistic programming practitioner in New York City, explained to me the clinical details of why repetition works. The upshot is that if you repeat the same action a minimum of five times, your brain will absorb the message and begin to form a new habitual behavior. If, for example, you have the habit of going downstairs and turning left when you get to the door, if you turn to the right instead, doing so will become familiar after you've done it five times. (Obviously it might take four or seven times, but you get the idea).

I can't tell you how many times I've heard business professionals say, "If your clients come back to you several times, by the fourth, they're yours." Do you always go to the same hair salon, even if your favorite hairdresser left long ago? It's easy to form a habit. You drive to the hair salon, park the car, check the new shoes in that shop on your walk there, and flip through magazines as you wait to be served.

I spend a lot of time with my clients finding substitute activities for eating because it can be tricky to find the one that they won't mind repeating until it sinks in and can overrule an emotional eating habit. The "prescription" is different for every person, too, and it may change over time. The Five-Times Method necessarily involves an activity that you find pleasurable or worthwhile. Remember, it's all too easy to make emotional eating habitual, because there's nothing much easier than putting something in your mouth. Your replacement activity shouldn't be a chore, unless it delivers consistent gratification.

Use Toothpaste, Mouthwash, or Gum

This might sound a little kooky, but it really works. There have been studies showing that children and adults with braces on their teeth often lose weight, because when they eat they know they have to spend a lot of time cleaning their braces, which is a boring chore (but better than facing the dentist's drill). They'd rather not snack if they know they have to spend a lot of annoying time getting the bits and bobs out of their teeth. Brushing your teeth will do more than make your dentist happy; it can actually improve your waistline.

Even if you don't have braces, you can brush your teeth or use mouthwash more often, and not just when you're finished eating. The act of brushing your teeth and the sweet taste of toothpaste may send a signal to your brain that the meal is over in much the same way a scoop of ice cream does. The scent can take your mind off food. The strong mint flavor has a suppressive effect on your taste buds, and the overpowering scent may take your mind off food. Remember, brushing is a habit for you already; it shouldn't be difficult to do it more frequently.

If you don't have a brush and toothpaste handy, try chewing a piece of strongly flavored mint gum or sucking on a sugar-free hard mint. I'm not a fan of chewing gum—I don't think all the chewing is good for your digestion or your colon—but each stick has only a few calories (or less if it's sugar free), and if the taste stops you from eating a whole lot more food, then it's certainly worth a try.

Use Your Friends

Lydia was by nature a very friendly and talkative person, and she found an ideal solution to breaking her emotional eating habit. Instead of eating when she was anxious, bored, or depressed, she would pick up the phone and call her friend Jody, who was equally chatty and had a great sense of humor. "I call Jody an *all-ogist*," Lydia told me with a laugh. "Because she always thinks she knows it all! So I would say to her, you know I want to sell my house and buy another one in the country, and she would take a deep breath and then go on and on about, well, what you have to do is this and then you have to do that and what about the money and what if you don't like the country after all and what about the language…and on and on. We would talk so much and she would make me laugh so much I would forget about eating!"

You might not need your own all-ogist (I'm not even sure that Jody's accepting clients!), but if you have a trusted and loving friend who understands what you're trying to do, who is supportive and helpful, make regular phone dates. Try to schedule him or her for the time of day when you are most likely to turn to food. Avoid the speaker function, though; you want to keep you hands on the phone and not on a fork!

Make Lists

Making a list can be very helpful, as it encourages you to think about courses of action. Consider this activity as an important step in your weight-loss journey.

The Boring List

This list isn't meant to put you to sleep. It's meant to keep you from *effectively* snoozing and giving in to mindless, emotional eating.

Write "The Boring List" at the top of the page. On one half of the paper write "When do I eat out of boredom?" On the other half of the paper write "What can I do instead?"

Take your time filling this out. Coming up with creative solutions that really work is the key. But if you're using your imagination, this shouldn't take too long: there are so many incredible things to see and do in this world that no one should ever be bored!

When do I eat out of boredom?	What can I do instead?
I don't have a date on Friday night.	Invite a friend to watch a movie
	Organize a poker game night

There doesn't need to be a single solution. Come up with as many as you can for each typical instance in which you'll fall back on emotional eating by default.

The Happiness List

This should be an open-ended list that includes everything you love in life that does *not* involve food. What is it that makes you happy? Write down at least ten things or activities, for example:

1. Window shopping
2. Taking long walks in the park
3. Reading a good book

Be sure that you include activities you can do at home as well. Since emotional eating is a nocturnal affair for many people, you should have at least a few "happy options" that don't require stepping outside. One friend of mine keeps copies of her favorite books and plays on her bedside table. She knows these works by heart, but they always appear fresh and delightful, and for her they're far better emotional relaxants than any food.

So Many Methods: Which Do I Choose?

Maybe you just read through these few suggestions for combating emotional eating and you're frowning. You think that nothing I mentioned could work. There's no boyfriend or best friend to call. The weather is lousy for walking. You don't like exercise. You don't like reading. The taste of mint makes you nauseous. Visiting your parents is an invitation to join World War III.

Fine. Then I assign you the task of making your own list, based on your own conditions. At the least, working on the list should distract you, momentarily, from the contents of a potato chip bag.

If you haven't yet found your antidote to emotional eating, keep thinking. Write down anything that sounds remotely interesting. Have you always wanted to learn how to surf? What about learning how to knit or sew? Have you ever wondered what it would be like to salsa? Write it down.

Be creative. Be honest. You will be amazed at what you come up with! Even if you never do these things, take some time to find out about them. That's a distraction in itself. And it may open you up to other, more feasible possibilities.

Some of the answers I've heard are amazing. One woman wanted to paint the outside of her house; another wanted to be a volunteer at the Salvation Army; another wanted to learn flamenco; yet another wanted to learn feng shui so she could get rid of all the accumulated junk in her garage and clear the energy in her home. On the first pass, none of these people had any idea that these activities might mean something to them. They had to clear their minds and focus on those empty, emotionally charged moments to come up with inspired solutions.

The point is that a simple list can be a catalyst for change. You've started the necessary, positive internal dialogue that will carry you from A to Z. You're thinking of alternatives to habits you know aren't good for you. You're wondering what else you can do to keep busy or add more joy and health into your world. You're planting the seeds in your garden of Alternatives to Emotional Eating. Some of them might sprout very quickly; others will need more time to germinate.

It is an amazingly empowering experience to come up with this list. You generate your own ideas of what can help improve your life. There is no right or wrong; it's whatever works for you. But whatever you decide, you need to *own* it. That's the only way your ideas can work.

Now, if you've done your lists and you're *still* overeating or eating foods that are unhealthy for you, this does not mean that you're a failure. All it means is that you need to keep working at it. You need to dig deeper into desires and interests you've long neglected. Eventually, you will uncover the methods and passions that will work best for you.

Summary

- *Emotional eating usually involves eating the comfort foods of childhood, foods high in sugar and carbohydrates.*

- *Emotional eating is caused by many factors such as anxiety, unhappiness, a desire to please others, and boredom.*

- *It's important to discover the root cause of your emotional eating as well as your eating personality in order to figure out a way to control it.*

- *Emotional eating is a habit that can be broken slowly and over time.*

- *There are many ways to break the habit of emotional eating, such as substituting unhealthy foods and behaviors with healthy ones; the Five-Times method; focusing your energy on something other than the unhealthy food you are craving, such as physical activity and nurturing relationships; and making lists. You need to find what works for you.*

Chapter Nine

YOU ARE WHAT YOU EAT

A t this stage, you know how to design your own nutritional plan. You know that sugar, unchecked, is an enemy to the *Yes, You Can* achievable diet. You've accepted that if you don't control your addiction, you will pile on pounds very quickly.

In addition:

* You know what type of personality eater you are and have embraced the role of the Decision Maker when it comes to your food.

* You've made no big announcements about your weight loss. and you're committed to taking one letter at a time in the process of the journey from A to Z.

* You've managed to break entrenched habits and embrace new ones. You do not feel annoyed when an old habit comes back because you accept that old habits resurface now and then. You know the process from A to Z is not a race down the road but more like a waltz or a leisurely stroll, and graciously you are moving forward. You feel calm.

* You are aware of what (and who) can sabotage your changes

* You've identified your emotional eating triggers and are compiling methods of dealing with them.

* You have an understanding of calories and their connection to your weight.

* You can design your own diet and lose as much weight you want.

What's in Your Food?

You're getting tantalizingly close to the Z. At the start of this book, I said that I want you to treat your body as a temple. Now that you are slimming down, it is very important for you to choose food that has excellent nutritional value and not just empty calories. Now, you're ready to wade into a few technicalities about what's actually in your food.

Almost all foods are mixtures of carbohydrates (starches and sugars), protein, fat, and water, along with an assortment of vitamins, minerals, and other nutrients. While some foods may have much more of one component than others, keep in mind that when we talk about a food as being a good source of a particular nutrient—protein, let's say—it also has other value. By the same token, a food that has a nutrient you seek can also be weighed down by lots of calories supplied by nutrients—say fat—you aren't crazy to have in abundance.

Nuts are the classic example of a hard bargain between great nutrition and big calories. They're full of protein, good dietary fat, fiber, and a few carbohydrates, as well as doses of calcium and potassium. What's not to love?

Well, look closely at a serving of almonds, for example. The suggested serving is one ounce (twenty-eight grams) or about twenty-five nuts, about as many as you fit in a large handful. Why so few? Because that handful contains about 170 calories, more than enough for a good snack. Unfortunately, it's all too easy to gobble a couple of handfuls; suddenly you're driving your calorie count way up.

A food that is good in small doses doesn't always supply unlimited returns in unlimited amounts. In the case of the almonds, too many means lots of calories, fat calories in particular, that hold you back from achieving your diet. Wishful thinking might tell you those extra calories somehow don't count, but they all count in the end.

To keep clear of such pitfalls, let's take a tour through the food components and up your awareness of how they work in your system.

Carbohydrates

Ah, the infamous carbs. This is a word you certainly know, and well you should. Carbohydrates dominate starchy, sugary foods such as grains, potatoes, beans, and of course, sugar. But almost all foods have some carbohydrates in them.

Milk, for instance, is fairly high in carbs because it contains lactose, a type of sugar. If you don't know this, your morning cup of coffee (or three) might become a small but substantial calorie pit (nonfat and whole milk have an equal amount of carbs). If you like a sweetener such as sugar or honey, the calorie pit gets deeper; add a caramel swirl or whipped cream on top, and you see why certain coffee chains are doing their share to hike carb counts worldwide.

When you digest carbohydrates, the starch or sugar is converted into glucose, the sugar that provides quick energy. That's usually a good thing, because you need that energy. In fact, if you're at a good weight and don't have any health problems, you can do just fine with carbs accounting for half your total calories. But if you're reading this book, you probably have weight to lose; in this condition carbs can pose real problems of both quantity and quality.

Carbohydrates fall into two basic classes: simple and complex. Simple carbohydrates are foods that have natural sugars, such as fruits, vegetables, milk, and dairy products. Refined grains such as white flour are also considered simple carbs. In moderation and as a solo act, simple carbs from natural sugars are fine. They add to diet problems, though, when they are made from refined grains and then blended with added sugars in products such as white bread, most breakfast cereals, snack foods, and so on. Highly processed foods with added sugars have far fewer nutrients than foods with natural sugars, and they usually have a lot more calories. These foods are also digested much more quickly, which can cause spikes in your blood sugar—so eating them may actually make you feel hungrier.

Quite often I hear people say, "I am losing weight because I am cutting down on refined sugar." My answer to that is "Not exactly. You are losing weight because you are cutting down on sugar, period—refined *and* not refined." This isn't criticism, of course. Cutting down on refined sugars is a great idea, but for those detoxing from sugar, it helps to know the extent of sugar's reach.

It also helps to understand the similarities between two foods: an apple and a chocolate chip cookie. Yes, they're both simple carbs, and like all carbs they pack four calories per gram. So the challenge is not to discover which food has more calories; rather, it's to discover which four calories are good and which are empty. If you're not quite prepared for making such distinctions, a good rule of thumb is that packaged foods probably aren't preferable to food in its natural state. Cookies often come in packages. Apples generally don't.

Complex carbohydrate foods generally are starchier and contain a lot of dietary fiber. These foods are good sources of energy, but while they, too, are converted to glucose and absorbed in the bloodstream, they are converted more slowly than simple carbs, without the sudden glucose spike. Whole grains, beans, corn, potatoes, and seeds are all good examples of complex carbohydrates. Because these foods are less processed, they're also good sources of micronutrients—vitamins and minerals—often removed by the refining process.

When you eat whole grain bread, for instance, you get more fiber, more nutrition, and more flavor than processed white bread can deliver, and the whole-grain bread has a less violent impact on your blood sugar. But remember, any carb has four calories per gram, so there's not much of a calorie difference between these breads. So while I strongly recommend substituting whole grains for processed grains, you still need to keep an eye on how much you eat. Whole-grain options are not always your friend. A whole-wheat jelly doughnut, for instance, is just as high in calories and almost as low in nutrition as one made with refined white flour.

Complex carbohydrates also contain dietary fiber—the indigestible part of plant foods. The fiber in these foods helps to slow their absorption into the blood, thereby playing a role in keeping your blood sugar under control.

How Many Carbs Should You Eat?

It's a great question, but it doesn't have a simple answer. Nutritionists might recommend you get anywhere from 45 to 65 percent of your daily calories from complex carbs. What would that twenty-point swing mean for your diet?

Let's imagine you've devised a 2,000-calorie daily diet. The conventional wisdom would suggest you consume 900 to 1,300 carb calories a day, or between 225 and 325 grams. For most of my weight-loss clients, though, those numbers are too high. The door is still open for lots of unwanted sugar and empty calories that encourage the consumption of yet *more* calories.

Each of my clients has found achievable methods for cutting back on carbs, especially the refined ones. Simple substitutions or changes in serving portions often do the trick: eating two helpings of broccoli and one of mashed potatoes at dinner, for instance. Berries, an apple, or a handful of nuts for a snack instead of cake will keep you satisfied by supplying a smaller amount of calories that pack in nutrition and are more satisfying than a larger number of empty calories.

Cutting back on carbs will be much easier if you're aware of how many of them you'll find in common foods. Here are a few basic, helpful guidelines:

* Meat, fish, cheese, and eggs have very few carbs.

* One slice of bread has, on average, about fifteen grams of carbs.

* One cup of cooked white rice has about forty-five grams carbs.

* One cup of cooked pasta has about forty grams carbs.

* Milk, no matter what the fat content, has twelve grams of carbs per eight-ounce cup.

* One cup of yogurt has about sixteen grams of carbs.

* One ounce of nuts has, on average, about five grams of carbs.

* Half a cup of cooked beans, any kind, has on average about twenty grams of carbs.

* One medium potato has about forty grams of carbs; ten french fries have about sixteen grams of carbs.

* One medium sweet potato has about twenty grams of carbs.

* Salad greens and leafy green vegetables generally have less than five grams carbs per serving.

* Starchier veggies, such as carrots and butternut squash, have between five and fifteen grams of carbs per serving.

* Strawberries are very low in carbs, under five grams per serving.

* One medium apple has twenty grams of carbs.

* One medium banana has twenty-eight grams of carbs.

* One medium orange has sixteen grams of carbs; eight ounces of orange juice have twenty-seven grams of carbs.

* Most other fruits have about ten grams of carbs per serving.

Estimating the carbs in processed foods and baked goods is very difficult, because these foods vary so much from manufacturer to manufacturer. As a basis for comparison, five chocolate crème sandwich cookies contain approximately fifty-five grams of carbohydrates. Read the food label on a box of cookies if you care to see what the carbs per serving are. One look should be enough; you may well be horrified to discover the extent that these foods are comprised of low-quality carb calories.

If there is no label (maybe you're dining out), it's safe to assume your food will be high in carbs if it's made with flour, potatoes, or sugary ingredients. That applies to a lot of popular menu items, including chicken dishes that featuring breading or sauces. Don't fall for the false virtue: "It's OK, chicken is low in carbs!" Yes it was, before it was covered in a sugar-laden glaze. The preparation may be delicious, but it can heap hidden carbs and lots of calories onto you meal.

Fiber for Fullness

While we were discussing carbs, fiber made a quick cameo appearance that might have caught your eye. It should have: adding fiber to your diet is key to achieving weight loss. A diet high in fiber is usually low in those processed foods with lots of added sugars. A high-fiber diet has fewer calories, more nutrition, and more satisfaction. It's rich in whole grains, fruits, vegetables, nuts, and legumes, which means it's rich in flavor, too.

Dietary fiber is the indigestible parts of plant foods. The fiber is what gives fruits and vegetables their crunch and chewiness. Fiber falls into two categories: insoluble and soluble. Insoluble fiber is mostly cellulose, the main fiber in the cell walls of all plant foods (think the stringy part of a celery stalk), and it doesn't dissolve in water. Soluble fiber does, and it forms a sort of soft gel in your intestines.

Both types of fiber hold water and help keep your bowels moving along smoothly, preventing constipation. It's likely that a high-fiber diet helps lower your blood cholesterol, and as I mentioned earlier, it helps keeps your blood sugar on an even keel.

Many foods have experienced wild swings of popularity among weight-loss experts, but the stock of high-fiber foods has remained consistently high. They literally aid the metabolic process from beginning to end. These foods help you feel full and keep your calorie counts low. And the body doesn't digest fiber; it passes right through, so it has no calories. Don't miss the key benefit here: if you substitute a high-fiber food for a high-calorie, processed one, you automatically cut back on your body's calorie count, even if the foods initially were calorically equal.

In my experience, most people aren't ingesting enough fiber. Most are getting by on less that twenty grams a day, a shortfall typical in Western diets that are dominated by processed foods. Thirty grams a day is more like it, and people with diabetes should aim to consume up to forty grams per day. Generally, you should be taking in fifteen grams of fiber for every one thousand daily calories.

Now, this doesn't mean you're restricted to an onslaught of bran and wheat germ unless that's what you actually like. Listing your preferred foods usually will yield some obvious opportunities to up the fiber and cut calories. For instance, instead of a glass of orange juice with zero fiber, why not have the whole orange? That would add three grams of fiber right there. It would also save a lot of calories. The juice has about one hundred calories, the orange only about forty-five.

When adding fiber in the form of vegetables, fruit, nuts, and so on, it's important to remember that these foods must *substitute* for other foods. A healthy diet will cut back on the refined, high-carb foods and replace them complex, high-fiber carbs. Remember the halo effect! Adding a big serving of broccoli to a burger and fries (with ice cream for dessert) doesn't do anything to reduce the unwanted calories. Magical thinking does not lead to better nutrition and weight loss!

Protein

Almost all of your body, except for your bones and teeth, is made up of protein. A protein is a complex, large molecule that's made up of strings of amino acids. And what are amino acids? They're the building blocks of protein, small molecules made up of atoms of hydrogen, oxygen, nitrogen, and carbon, with a bit of sulfur here and there. Humans need just twenty-two different amino acids to build the many thousands of different proteins that make up the body. Just as we use the alphabet to put together words and then string those words into sentences, your body uses amino acids to string together the proteins that keep you alive.

The amino acids fall into two categories: essential and nonessential. There are nine essentials, and the only way for you to get them is to eat them. The rest of the amino acids, the nonessential, are compounds based on the nine essentials.

Great, you might say. Now, where do I get these essential acids? Simple: from food that already contains protein. Animal-based foods, such as meat, eggs, fish, and dairy, contain all the essential amino acids. That's why nutritionists call them complete or high-quality proteins.

Plant foods also contain amino acids but are considered incomplete proteins because they don't contain *all* the essential amino acids. Beans, nuts, and whole grains are better as protein sources, but they're also usually lacking in one or more of the essential amino acids.

Corn, for example, is low on the essentials tryptophan and cysteine. This explains why eating mostly corn and no animal products would quickly leave you malnourished. Fortunately, vegetarians can select from a wide variety of plant foods to collect all the essential amino acids. But this requires some education and thought; it's easy for vegetarians to eat a great many carbs—and therefore sugar—if they aren't selective. This is why many people who are looking to cut carbs prefer a diet that includes at least some animal products: more protein, fewer carbs.

The formulas for figuring that out the proper amount of dietary protein are complex; generally, they come down to 0.36 grams of protein for every pound of body weight. If you weigh 140 pounds, then your daily protein needs come to about 50 grams a day. A gram of protein is four calories, so that means you would need only about two hundred calories a day from protein to maintain good health, probably about 10 to 15 percent of your daily calories. As a general rule, men need more protein than women, mostly because men are larger and have more muscles. If you're an athlete or bodybuilder, your protein needs might be slightly higher—but you don't need to force down protein shakes and supplements. Adding a couple of egg whites a day or having slightly larger meat portions should provide you with all the extra protein you might need.

In our society, it's very, very easy to get your basic protein requirement and then some. Even vegetarians get about fifty to one hundred grams of protein a day, and people who eat meat get much more. It comes back to portion sizes. A baked chicken leg, for instance, has about thirty grams of protein. Eat two, and you've already exceeded your minimum protein needs for the day. A chicken egg, which has the ideal balance of all the essential amino acids, has six grams of protein. A glass of milk has eight grams. On the plant food side, an ounce of cashews has four grams of protein, while half a cup of cooked kidney beans has nearly eight grams and a cup of cooked brown rice has five. Just a quarter-cup serving of tofu, or soybean curd, contains nearly thirteen grams of protein.

So never mind the protein-proud steak eaters; vegetarians and vegans can hit their daily protein needs without consuming any animal products at all.

Because your protein need is only 10 percent of your daily calories, you should sense an opportunity to cut some calories from your diet via more substitutions. A four-ounce serving of steak, for example, gives you thirty-four grams of protein and about two hundred calories. That's most of the protein you need for the day, which means you can cut back on steak and add lower-calorie vegetables and legumes (that will round out the protein ration) and still receive quality nutrition.

Fat

This is where you might encounter serious confusion, and I don't blame you. Conventional wisdom rails against fat, fat and more fat; meanwhile, what's the substance you're trying to melt off your thighs and waistline? I have to expect a little cognitive dissonance if I announce that fat is good and that the body needs it. And sure enough, most people hear that and are astonished. If you are, too, join the crowd.

The confusion over fat comes from mixing up excess body fat, which is why people come to me in the first place, with fat in the diet. It's made worse by advertising and confusing medical advice about the value of low-fat foods and a low-fat diet. And it is true that a gram of fat contains nine calories, more than twice as much as a gram of carbohydrates or protein.

Let's try to clear up the confusion. You need fat in your diet. Fat is a source of quick energy. You need it to absorb vitamins A, D, E, and K. Your body uses fat to make cell membranes, hormones, neurotransmitters, and more. You need some fat in your body to keep you warm, to cushion your organs, to store energy against times of scarcity or an illness, and to keep your joints well oiled.

Just as you need essential amino acids from your food in order to build all the different proteins your body needs, you also need essential fatty acids for building the twenty different fatty acids that are the foundation of cell membranes, all your body's hormones, and other chemical messengers. If you don't eat enough dietary fat, you won't get enough essential fatty acids for good health.

The two essential fatty acids are linoleic acid and linolenic acid. It's almost impossible to keep them separate with such similar names, so it might help to refer to these acids by their more popular monikers. Linoleic acid, which is an important component of many oils, is known as omega-6 fatty acid (never mind the reason why; it's too complicated to explain here). Linolenic acid, which is found in marine and plant oils, is called omega-3 fatty acid.

Omega-6 fatty acids are found in most cooking oils, including corn, sunflower, safflower, and soybean. They also occur in nuts and seeds: walnuts, almonds, sunflower seeds, and peanuts are all good sources.

Omega-3s are found in cold-water fish such as salmon, tuna, and herring, in the leaves and seeds of many plants, and in egg yolks. Good plant sources of omega-3s are nuts, soybeans, canola oil, and flaxseed.

Omega-3 fatty acids are essential to life, and they also can lower your cholesterol, bring down high blood pressure, and help prevent strokes and heart attacks. The best amount for optimal health seems to be roughly one gram a day. That's not that hard to get. One 3.5-ounce serving of canned salmon, for instance, has 3 grams; a serving of canned tuna has about 1.5 grams. There are about 500 milligrams of omega-3s in a gram of flaxseed oil.

Omega-9 fatty acid (also called oleic acid) is the fatty acid found in olive oil, peanut oil, avocados, and nuts. Omega-9 fatty acids aren't, de facto, essential. But it's hard for me, with my French and Italian grandmothers, to imagine a kitchen without olive oil. Many nutritionists believe that the liberal use of olive oil is one reason the traditional Mediterranean diet is so healthful. Olive oil seems to play a role in heart health, stroke prevention, and keeping your blood pressure down.

Saturated vs. Unsaturated vs. Trans Fats: Whom Do You Love?

On one hand, the difference between saturated and unsaturated fats is simply chemical. Saturated fats, which are found mostly in animal foods such as lard and butter, are solid at room temperature. Unsaturated fats—all of which are either monounsaturated or polyunsaturated—are liquid at room temperature (think cooking oils). But on the other hand, their interactions with the human body are markedly different.

Diets high in saturated fats have gotten a lot of bad press in recent years, since there's a growing body of evidence linking them to high blood cholesterol and increased risk of heart disease and stroke. But both monounsaturated fats (like olive, canola, and peanut oils) and polyunsaturated fats (fish, flaxseed, corn, and sunflower seed oil) may actually *lower* cholesterol and help *prevent* heart disease. In small amounts saturated fats are fine, but if you prefer them you probably should be careful about how often you use them.

There's only one fat that should be avoided at all costs (unless you're into a free meal). Partially hydrogenated vegetable oil, also known as trans fats, gets the worst press of all, and for good reason. Trans fats are perfectly good vegetable oils that have been processed to the point where they, like saturated fats, are solid at room temperature. They're lurking in margarine, baked goods, potato chips, and other manufactured foods that are pretty much bad news across the board.

Since trans fats have been linked to diabetes, heart disease, cancer, and a lot of other serious health issues, consumer pressure has forced food manufacturers to cut back on their use, yet they're still all over the market. Read the labels carefully and avoid them. If in fact you do have too much fat in your diet, these are the fats to target for elimination.

"Low Fat" = Low Quality

When the war on fat began, food manufacturers quickly got wise and exploited people's worries by offering low-fat versions of traditionally high-fat foods. These "healthy" options are still out there in most food outlets: entrees, desserts, and snacks of all kinds in low-fat form being marketed as a healthy choice.

If you fall for this marketing regularly, you can expect your weight loss to grind to a full stop. Unfortunately, these low-fat options usually have just as many calories as the full-fat version. To make these products palatable, additional ingredients—often just more sugar or other sweeteners—are pumped in, along with a false sense of virtue. *Great,* you think, *they're low fat! I can eat more than before!* And so it goes: bigger portion, more calories (mostly of the low-quality variety), more of your daily calorie needs met before you get to the healthy foods. Weight gain is all too easy. Sugar addiction awaits.

If you can't do without some cookies or potato chips, I recommend that you buy the full-fat version. Hopefully, you can train yourself to eat a smaller portion and find greater satisfaction.

Vitamins and Minerals

Last but not least, let's talk about vitamins and minerals, the remaining essential building blocks for living.

Vitamins and minerals are both essential to normal bodily function, but very small doses are needed. Vitamins are organic substances; minerals are nonorganic. Ideally, you'll receive all your vitamins and minerals from your diet, but supplements are a legitimate option.

There are thirteen vitamins and about a dozen important minerals. There are plenty of excellent books and Web sites that explain their chemical importance in detail; in this book I'll simply discuss how you can get sufficient doses of them and what dietary changes you might make to achieve a compete nutritional plan.

Fruits, vegetables, whole grains, and nuts are all rich sources of the essential vitamins and minerals. If your diet includes plenty of these foods, you're probably getting all the vitamins and minerals you need for good health without even trying. There are some exceptions, though.

The B vitamins, such as folic acid, niacin, and thiamin, are found only in animal products: meat, poultry, fish, eggs, and dairy foods. If you're a strict vegetarian or vegan, you might not be getting enough Bs, especially vitamin B12. As we get older, we can't absorb the B vitamins from our food as well as we used to. And if you're a woman of childbearing age, it's crucial to get sufficient folic acid from your diet to help prevent birth defects.

Your skin absorbs sunlight to manufacture vitamin D. Small amounts occur naturally in eggs, and vitamin D also is added to milk and a few other foods, like orange juice. If you're a shut-in, or living at a high latitude, the lack of sunlight might lead to a vitamin D deficiency if your diet doesn't compensate.

Calcium is essential to bone growth and health, and aids in many other crucial functions. It's most abundant in dairy foods; people who avoid dairy need to take deliberate steps to make sure they aren't calcium deficient.

One reason I encourage you to check in with your physician before you begin my program is because it's important to detect any existing nutritional deficiencies through blood work. You might be lacking iron, which can cause tiredness and anemia. Diabetics often are low on potassium and magnesium, and vitamin D deficiency isn't uncommon in the general population. Serious deficiencies require medical help for correction; more often, the condition is mild and can be remedied through dietary changes or by introducing an over-the-counter supplement.

It's easy to worry about reaching your recommended daily allowance for all these substances, but if you make a few positive changes in your diet you'll likely increase your doses of vitamins and minerals, even if you're eating fewer calories. When you achieve weight loss in part by substituting quality foods for old, empty-calorie choices, your overall nutrition improves. Nuts and whole grains, for instance, are good sources of calcium, iron, magnesium, zinc, and vitamin E. But don't forget to keep those portions under control!

The Glycemic Index

Originally the glycemic index (GI) wasn't a tool for weight loss at all. Rather, it helped people manage diabetes, prediabetes, or blood sugar problems through diet. That said, it's also true that foods that are low on the glycemic index tend to be low in calories.

If you need to keep an eye on your blood sugar, the glycemic index is very useful. But if you simply want to lose weight while still eating a varied and nutritious diet, the index can sharpen your nutritional IQ and help you make better overall food choices. Either way, you should know how it works.

The GI is a way to measure how quickly a carbohydrate food is converted to glucose and absorbed into your bloodstream. The GI uses white sugar as a baseline; since it is 100 percent carbohydrate, white sugar scores 100. Eat a spoonful of it, and it will be converted to glucose in your blood almost at once. In contrast, the carbs in a serving of kidney beans will be converted to blood sugar much more slowly; on the GI, kidney beans are ranked at 23. The GI rates kidney beans as an excellent vehicle for carbohydrates if you're cautious about blood-sugar spikes. Meanwhile, foods with high GI values almost always contain high doses of refined carbs that are absorbed into the bloodstream quickly, sometimes much too quickly. Complex carbs, such as those found in beans, make a much less dangerous impact.

How do the low GI index foods work their magic? Good old fiber is a big factor; it slows down digestion generally, including the rate at which the carbs are processed. The type of starch in a high-carb food also is a factor. Starch, a new player in your diet IQ, comes in three varieties: rapidly digestible, which hits your bloodstream within 20 minutes; slowly digestible, which takes between 20 and 120 minutes; and resistant starch, which can't even be digested in the small intestine. Like fiber, resistant starch passes through you without being absorbed and has no calories. Beans and lentils are naturally high in resistant starch. So are whole grains. Cooked potatoes and pasta are also high in resistant starch—but only after they've cooled and the starch has undergone chemical changes. The higher a food is in resistant starch, the lower it ranks on the GI.

So choosing these resistant starch foods will give you that special carb-satisfaction for a few less calories than the charts indicate. As a rule of thumb, any food with a GI rank below 60 is a good choice: it's likely high in vitamins, minerals, and fiber, low in calories, and it won't put undue stress on your blood sugar. Of course, the old caveat—don't overdo it!—applies; a low GI rank is no reason to eat too much of these foods, or any other.

High GI foods might have been fiber-rich once, but fiber can be removed. That's what happens when whole foods are processed (they lose most of their other nutrients as well). The more highly processed a food is, the higher the GI rank. The smaller the starchy particles in the food (think McDonald's hamburger rolls instead of grainy pumpernickel bread), the faster the carbs are absorbed.

Remember, the glycemic index applies only to foods that contain carbohydrates. Most vegetables are very low in carbs and rank 0 on the GI scale, including avocado, broccoli, cabbage, cauliflower, cucumber, green beans, and leafy greens, such as chard, kale, salad greens, and spinach.

This is a GI primer. If you are diabetic or simply would like more information, there are abundant online sources that explain the glycemic value of foods.

Fad Diets

Like the glycemic index, other tools created for medical purposes are being incorporated into fads as well. For instance, a gluten-free diet eliminates anything made with wheat and aides people with celiac disease, who must restrict their gluten intake. But "gluten-free" is a popular trend now; you might have noticed, since the phrase is being used to sell yet more processed foods.

I don't recommend banning gluten unless there's a medical necessity. It's far too restrictive for good health on a long-term basis. Not only that, you may well *gain* weight instead of losing it.

The Cost of Better Nutrition

I can't tell you how often someone has moaned to me, "But, Diana, it's so expensive to eat better!" I'm certainly sensitive to financial issues. But is it really more expensive to eat healthier food and sustain a sensible diet?

A little, perhaps, but not a lot. If you compare the cost of a family-size bag of pretzels, for instance, to the cost of half a dozen peaches, the pretzels are cheaper. This type of one-for-one, superficial comparison always seems to favor the processed foods.

But once you've moved your nutritional IQ into a high gear, you'll see there's more to the story than the price tag. How far does the food go? What does it deliver in terms of dietary needs?

You can eat half the bag of pretzels at one sitting, ingesting 700 or more calories that are empty, or nearly so. You might eat three peaches in a row, but you'll only be getting about 150 calories and much more in the way of nutrition. Which food, really, is more expensive? Which is the better overall value?

Stopping at the grocery store on the way home from work and buying one of the good prepared meals (rotisserie chicken, mashed potatoes, some veggies, a bag of premade salad) is more expensive than taking everyone to KFC. But it's almost as convenient and a much better choice from a nutritional perspective. When you're mindfully eating good foods, you need less of them to feel satisfied. Two portions equal in weight are not equal in dietary value.

I hear a lot of complaints about the cost of prepared "diet" foods. A frozen dinner from a company that specializes in weight-control options is indeed more expensive than a brand that's not portion controlled (although these aren't exactly cheap). But the fact that one brand gives you more food, yet costs less, should tell you everything you need to know about its nutritional quality. Subsisting on low-quality foods often results in back-end payments—and bad health—that don't get mentioned by the marketers.

I'm actually a fan of frozen dinners in a pinch. There are times when you simply don't have the time or energy to cook something for yourself. The temptation to order in a large pizza or stop by a fast-food chain is ever present.

But if you have a low-sodium, low-fat, portion- controlled dinner in the freezer, you can avoid the fast food and still have a quick, satisfying meal. I'm sure you can guess that I don't recommend that you subsist on frozen dinners. However, a world of long workdays, tight budgets, and demanding family schedules requires a few coping mechanisms. A low-calorie frozen option on the toughest days is far from a deal breaker.

A family trip to the fast-food franchise isn't the end of the world, either. If that's all you have time for, there's a simple means to stay within your dietary range: order from the dollar or children's menu. You'll get a small burger, small fries, maybe a salad and a diet drink. It's hardly ideal, but you at least can keep the portion under control. Remember, the new standard meal sizes were not created with high nutritional IQ in mind!

Cooking to Cut Costs

But here's a radical idea: if you fear the influence of frozen dinners and fast foods (or you're bored by them, even better!), why not cook more? There simply isn't a better way to save money and ensure your family has good nutrition with a lot of variety.

A lot of my clients groan when I suggest this (except for the ones who phone their personal chefs to tell them they'll be home for dinner more often). They don't really know how to cook—their experience in the kitchen seems to be limited mostly to reheating things in the microwave. Some of them literally don't know how to turn on their ovens. They think of cooking as something that's beyond them, or as a chore that requires a huge amount of boring work. Some have teenagers who greet them in the evening by clamoring to be fed. Cooking just seems daunting.

I could begin by explaining that cooking will save you money, create easy leftover meals for later in the week, put portion control under your control, and literally bring your family around the table and give them satisfaction, once they see that creating inventive, delicious, and healthy food isn't a magical art. But I'll start with a simpler message: cooking is fun.

When I take on a client who insists she or he can't cook, I set up a lunch meeting. I prepare a great meal while we talk, and we still have plenty of time to enjoy it before the session is over. Watching me prepare a simple, delicious, nutritious lunch with reasonable yet very satisfying portions makes these clients much more receptive to the good news about cooking.

Even though you and I can't arrange this, there are ways to learn that don't even require leaving your house. Of course, you can enroll in a local cooking class; these are getting very popular as more and more people realize they need these basic survival skills. But on YouTube you'll find thousands of great videos that demonstrate everything from how to boil water to preparing a roast turkey. You can also check out the many Web sites that offer basic recipes and videos.

Quite often, cooking is no more complex than applying enough heat to cook your food but not so much that you set the kitchen on fire. Beyond that, anything goes. Let your creativity out.

One of my favorite dinners for beginners starts with buying a whole-wheat pizza crust and good organic tomato sauce. Spread the sauce on the crust and turn on the oven. While it heats up, clean out the fridge. Whatever stragglers you find, throw them on the pizza: drooping veggies, cheese, pineapple, whatever suits your fancy. Put the pizza into the oven until the crust is crisp and the cheese is melted. Total prep time is about half an hour. Your fridge is cleaner, you've got minimal cleanup, and you've eaten well: What more can you ask?

Once you get the idea, start checking out cookbooks. Skip the expensive, all-color books by celebrity chefs. When these fellows cook in their restaurants, they've got a couple of sous chefs, a saucier, and a human dishwasher at their disposal. The home versions of their recipes are going to need expensive ingredients and more time and patience than you probably have. (Jacques Pepin, who has created recipes that truly do take time, space, and everyday ingredients into consideration, is an exception.)

Look for practical cookbooks that teach you techniques along with the recipes. They'll use lots of familiar, easy-to-find ingredients and simple methods with equipment you probably own. Plenty of them take your busy schedule into account and cut out unnecessary steps. There are literally dozens of great meals you can plate in less than thirty minutes.

Organic or Not?

I strongly recommend buying organically grown produce and meats whenever possible. Unfortunately, cost can be more of a factor here—organic products, particularly meats, are usually more expensive. They can also be inconvenient; the selection of organic products is usually small compared to the stock of conventionally grown produce.

But if you're taking achievable diet steps and you want to increase your knowledge of weight loss and health, organic foods will be hard to ignore. Once you've come to rely more heavily on fresh fruits and vegetables for nutrition, you probably won't relish being exposed to all the pesticides that are used on conventionally grown produce.

It's helpful, then to know about the "dirty dozen" and the "clean fifteen." These lists, compiled by the nonprofit Environmental Working Group in the US (www.ewg.org), round up the fruits and vegetables that, when conventionally grown, absorb the most pesticides and those that come to market relatively clean. You can save money by sticking to the clean fifteen and avoiding the higher organic price tags. If you buy any of the dirty dozen items that aren't organic, you can still reduce your pesticide exposure by rinsing all fruits and vegetables thoroughly and peeling those with thicker skins.

The Dirty Dozen

celery
peaches
strawberries
apples
blueberries
nectarines
bell peppers
spinach
cherries

kale/collard greens

potatoes

grapes

The Clean Fifteen

onions

avocado

corn

pineapple

mangos

peas

asparagus

kiwi

cabbage

eggplant

cantaloupe

watermelon

grapefruit

sweet potato

honeydew melon

Spoil Your Appetite?

In the introduction of this book, you read about my French grandmother, who encouraged me to "spoil my appetite." Meanwhile, my Italian *nonna* was appalled to find me snacking. "Don't spoil your appetite," she'd cry.

So, many clients and life experiences later, whose advice do you think I took?

All love and respect to Nonna, but I always say to clients, "Go ahead, spoil your dinner."

Eat five times a day. Three meals and two snacks. But feel free to take a quick bite of something healthy if it comes your way.

Nonna, along with many other loving mothers, fathers, and kitchen devotees, embraced a certain value system: the meal ravenously consumed is the one that's best enjoyed. Well, perhaps on a primal level it's true. But for people who want to retain control over what they eat and love food on their own terms (not the food's terms or a saboteur's), "going animal" at mealtimes just isn't great advice.

When you eat many times a day, you're inclined to take smaller portions at any one meal. I always make very sure to spoil my appetite before going out to dinner, especially when it's a business affair. If I turn up for the business meal feeling hungry, I feel like getting up on the table and eat everything on it—not very elegant. What's worse is if I'm that hungry, I'll say yes to anything just so I can get to the food. That's not the best way to do business. By spoiling my appetite before I leave for the dinner, I can put my knife and fork down during the meal and actually pay attention to the deal we're discussing. (Of course, I simultaneously hope that the people I'm negotiating with didn't spoil their appetites and will, out of sheer hunger, say yes to anything I propose!)

When I say spoil your appetite, by now you should realize that this means opting for good choices, not *any* choice. Spoiling a good dinner with a doughnut or french fries on the way home is spoilage through and through.

What I advocate is preparation for those hunger pangs that arise in the middle of the morning and the afternoon, during the long stretches between established mealtimes. And instead of ignoring them—out of some notion of virtue—give in and get some good nutrition, along with an energy boost that will sustain you until the meal. You'll sit down to lunch or dinner comfortably in the hunger two or hunger three zone: ready to enjoy what's there, but not desperate. This is mindful eating with more room for good choices that keep your calorie counts low.

Fresh fruit, along with a handful of nuts, is a great snack that can be enjoyed most anywhere; bananas in particular are filling, inexpensive, and easy to store and eat. Prepackaged string cheese is also a good choice. The various types of snack bars can be good options, but read the ingredients carefully, and check the calories. Some breakfast, trail mixes, and protein bars are really nothing but candy bars is disguise.

Last but First: Eat Breakfast

Many clients have told me that they skip breakfast to save calories. I rolled my eyes. "Why are you here?" I sometimes asked if they seem particularly self-righteous.

These people, many of them very overweight, eat nothing when they wake up and, lo and behold, are starving by ten a.m. They're at work, and what's to be found? Doughnuts and bagels in the break room. Coffee with sugar and creamers. Sadly, it's a common, low–nutritional IQ method of starting the day.

Enjoying a satisfying breakfast every morning is yet another example of how eating more can help you weigh less. If you leave the house feeling full, you'll eat less when it's time for a coffee break or lunch. You won't be so hungry that you grab the first thing in sight. Instead, you'll take the time to make good choices and eat more mindfully.

According to the National Weight Control Registry (www.nwcr.ws) in the US, people who eat breakfast every day are the most likely to not only lose a lot of weight but also keep it off in the long term.

Maybe you really *aren't* hungry when you wake up. You may well have spoiled your appetite by eating late the night before (and if so, I'll bet you snacked late to compensate for not eating enough during the day, including yesterday's breakfast!). Whatever the cause, if you don't feel hungry in the morning, make sure that you never eat after dinner; by sunrise, you'll have gone nearly twelve hours without food, and the thought of not "breaking fast" will be abhorrent. You'll want breakfast then.

"Midnight snacks" can become a seductive habit. It can be awfully comforting to have a cookie or two before bed to tide you over into pleasant dreams. But your body doesn't need to eat right before you go to sleep; you may feel a psychological yearning, but that's not the same thing at all (it's more emotional eating). Your body won't expend as much energy asleep as it does when you're awake and moving around. This is one situation in which it pays to listen to your body; its rhythms and needs should take precedence over the needs of your mind.

A good breakfast is like any other good meal. Aim for a flavorful mix of carbs, protein, and fat, and throw in some fresh fruit if possible. Be very conscious about portions and especially sugar intake—read the labels on your packages.

I've found that breakfast provides a greater challenge to weight loos than any other meal: people are more resistant to changes in this part of the day than any other. So again, proceed slowly. Makes small changes, but stick with them. Take the time for the changes to feel natural to you. Remember that you aren't trying simply to lose weight: you are building new habits that, with small adjustments, can last a lifetime.

In your daily A-to-Z process, breakfast sets the tone. So do the minimum: think of your breakfast as A, as in *apple*, and eat one!

Summary

- *An empty calorie is one that contains very little nutrients for the body and should be avoided when possible.*

- *It's important to understand the components and nutritional value of the food you're eating and create a healthy balance between carbohydrates, protein, fats, and fiber.*

- *An eating plan rich in fiber is a key to an achievable weight-loss plan.*

- *Eat organic whenever possible.*

- *Cooking simply can be easy, save you money, and be more nutritious— but if you must eat frozen dinners and/or fast food, it's still possible to make healthier food choices.*

- *Spoil your appetite—avoid becoming too hungry, which can lead to over-eating and poor food choices.*

- *Eat a balanced breakfast every morning.*

Chapter Ten

YES, YOU MUST EXERCISE
FOR WEIGHT LOSS

I know that some of you were hoping you'd get through this book without encountering this chapter. There are always a few of us who believe that the human body can get along fine as the modern world caters to our needs. Cars, public transport, escalators, elevators, and desk jobs are all a blessing. Aren't they all proof of human evolution?

Perhaps. But the human body hasn't accepted the blessing just yet. It's built to move and keep moving. Every system, every fiber of your being—yes, even cognitive function—is dependent on regular exercise for good health and prime function.

Our thinking has made great progress through the centuries, but our brains remain part of an organization that thrives when it receives good nutrition and plenty of oxygen and sags when it doesn't.

You've read nine chapters and learned a great deal about nutrition. Now it's time to accept the fact that the best nutrition in the world will do little good if it isn't burned efficiently, or if the body isn't supplied with enough oxygen. That fact holds up whether you're five, twenty-five, or ninety; if humans advance until they're mostly hanging around to age 140, it will hold up then, too.

When it comes to losing weight, you should think of exercise and proper nutrition as a set of hands. Just about any job you undertake will go more smoothly if you put both hands to use. People who neglect one hand or the other are going to have trouble eventually. You can exercise like you're crazy, but if you try to keep in training shape by living off snack cakes and alcohol, your body will stage a revolt (as I found out when I tried to make a go of the Nutella diet).

Conversely, you can engineer the purest, best balanced diet yet known to humanity, but if you think this will give you free license to sit at your desk by day and in front of your flat screen TV by night, the atrophy of your muscles (and yes, your brain) will be inevitable. I don't mind saying that I'd find this life, however long it lasted, intolerable. Once you've experienced the benefits and joy that can accompany regular exercise, it will be the same for you.

Move, Move, Move, Aerobically

By now, I'm sure you've incorporated a little more exercise into your daily life. Maybe you're climbing the stairs to your apartment instead of taking the elevator (going down the stairs, although not as taxing on your breathing, also burns plenty of calories). You walk to work when you can, take strolls after dinner in pleasant weather, or even stand up when you make phone calls instead of sitting down. Maybe you take the dog out for an extra run around the block in the evening. It's all great improvement, and each new effort pushes you a little closer toward the Z.

But now that I've applauded, I have to be clear: on their own, these little steps will never be enough keep you on the other side of your weight-loss finish line. To attain the lasting, powerful benefits of exercise, you really need to push a little harder, literally. You have to get some aerobic exercise every week.

I'm not going to start clamoring that you join a gym at once. Let's face it, for some of us, gyms are horribly boring places. Treadmills mean dreariness. Maybe you find this kind of exercise to be unnatural; humans didn't evolve in gyms, now did they? But even if you are proudly in this camp, you've got to come up with some method of raising your metabolic rate on a regular basis. Your list of choices is practically endless, so there will be no excuse.

Your chosen activities should boost your heart rate, accelerate your breathing, and raise your metabolic rate for at least half an hour. Those are the only requirements. Everything else is negotiable: where you exercise, how you do it, what muscles you engage, whether you're taking a break from work, playing morning tennis, or tangoing with joy (yes, many people have a *lot* of fun raising their metabolic rate).

Instead of going into the physiological details of just how elevated your metabolic rate should be during your exercise, you can run a simple test. I call it the "talking business threshold." While you're engaged in your workout, imagine that an important business call comes in. You pick up the phone (probably your cell, but you can exercise aerobically in the office if you have some privacy and/or tolerant coworkers!). How well are the words coming out?

If your breathing still allows you to talk normally, you aren't exercising hard enough. You should be panting. We're not talking about pushing to the brink of exhaustion, but your heart should be bumping in your chest, and speaking clearly should be difficult, if not impossible. Once you've got your metabolic rate up to an appropriate level, you shouldn't be conducting any business until you're finished exercising. Your delivery should be more appropriate for an obscene phone call than a quarterly report!

There are heart rate monitors and online calculators galore that can help you determine what level of exertion is appropriate for your weight and age. But the main thing to remember is that the exercise should be vigorous, not violent. It should be taxing, but not to the point where it's literally difficult to breathe. The level of exercise that's healthy for you is another subject that you should cover with your doctor before you engage in any weekly program.

Running Steps, to What End?

What, in a nutshell, are you trying to accomplish? Why is it so important to weight loss to raise your metabolic rate on a regular basis?

First of all, remember that you need to burn about 3,500 calories more than you ingest to lose a pound. The most stubborn fat on your body, which piled up in your abdominal area, can't be dislodged without regular aerobic exercise.

You've figured out how you can make modest, sometimes imperceptible cuts in your diet that will lower your caloric intake. But how wonderful would it be if you could *accelerate* the gap between what you take in and what you burn? That's where exercise comes in.

Money in the Bank

Here's a point where it's helpful to make a comparison between exercise and money. When you spend less than you make each month, you watch your assets literally growing. That creates a tremendously reassuring feeling. It tells you that you're living responsibly and keeping track of your spending.

But more money saved also means better interest rates on loans, more money for retirement, a higher credit score, and bundles set aside for emergencies. Saving money delivers benefits for the short and the long term; you'll be surprised to find how friendly loan officers can be when you've been saving consistently for a few years—and well they might be, since they make use of your money in the meantime!

Well, exercise helps your body in a similar way. Your body receives the short-term benefit of burning extra calories, which makes your immediate weight-loss goals all the more attainable. But regular exercise also makes the body more efficient. Once it's accustomed to regular exercise, your body naturally will burn more calories even while it's at rest. This is what is it means to *increase your metabolism.*

When it comes to your weight-loss goals, increasing your metabolism is the equivalent of running downhill. The trip to Z will be a great deal quicker if you can combine your high nutritional IQ with sensible and regular workouts.

Long-Range Returns

Not motivated yet? Maybe you don't believe that exercise is as wonderful as everyone says it is. After all, hype is everywhere: gyms need members, personal trainers need clients, and the sports equipment business has big, big profits to protect. If people stop exercising, a large chunk of our economy will sputter.

Well, this is one instance where there's not just smoke but plenty of fire. No matter how big a business fitness is, it's still essential to the health of every living person, including you. Your metabolism, in one sense, *is* a fire, and the more oxygen it receives via exercise, the more efficiently it burns fuel.

But let's quickly run down some of the reasons, beyond your waistline, that exercise is a body's best friend:

* Muscle maintenance. I'm not talking about building up bulging biceps and thighs of steel, unless those bragging rights really will motivate you. Much more important is maintenance of your core muscles, which help you get through the most basic movements in the course of your day, movements so automatic you probably take them for granted. The core muscles wrap around your torso and pelvic areas, and they're essential to maintaining good posture and back strength as you age.

* Endurance. Sure, you're going to be tired after you start exercising (you'll probably sleep wonderfully well on nights after a workout, another perk). But over time, as your body becomes ever more efficient, you'll be able to exercise longer and harder with ease, and the daily chores won't seem so taxing.

* Clean out the pipes. High-density lipoprotein, otherwise known as the "good" cholesterol, builds up when you exercise, while levels of low-density lipoprotein—the "bad" stuff —decrease. The upshot is cleaner arteries, which in turn dramatically reduce the risk of heart disease, stroke, and other serious issues that a balanced diet and exercise are engineered to avoid.

* Increased brain function. "Stop right there," the cynics will say. "I know exercise is great and all, but you're telling me it will make me *smarter*?"

* Yes, it is, and yes, it will. As John Medina, developmental molecular biologist and author of the best-selling *Brain Rules*, explains, the evidence is overwhelming that exercise is essential to peak cognitive function. Exercise increases the flow of oxygen to all parts of the body, and the brain thrives on oxygen. Studies have shown that older adults who exercise outperform their sedentary peers in tests of cognitive function; that's the short term. Long

term, exercise may decrease a person's chance of succumbing to dementia or Alzheimer's disease by as much as 50 percent. It turns out you might only be as smart as your metabolism.

* More efficient burn rate even at rest. Have you ever watched long-distance runners after they cross the line? Notice how they stand, then pace, panting all the while. That's a reward for the exercise: even at rest, their bodies continue to burn the calories at an accelerated rate. The more you exercise, the more you'll burn off in the aftermath of exercise. It's yet another example of residual payments on a deposit!

* And don't forget the weight loss. The importance of regular, sustained aerobic activity in an A-to-Z plan simply can't be overstated. It's often said that the more you know, the more you want to know. By the same principle, the more a body moves, the more it wants to move. Movement actually becomes easier, and that's half of your challenge right there.

* The results of slimming down and toning up with also feel delicious. If you simply cut calories, you'd never experience the joy of moving about in a toned body. Without exercise, you may feel cranky as you continue along your weight-loss journey, and as you should know by now, I believe your positive attitude is critical to success. Well, this is positive attitude in a workout: exercise makes you look *and* feel good.

Once at Bloomingdale's, in New York City, a striking woman passed me by too quickly for me to see her face. Yet I could tell that she was brimming with confidence and health: her posture was straight and true, her movements quick, supported by a good, muscular frame. Her clothes fell easily over her natural, attractive curves. From her pace, carriage, and hair (which showed some gray amidst the blond) I guessed that she was in her middle thirties and at most forty-five.

I circled around the woman quickly so that I could walk past her. She wore glasses over her gently tanned features. She clearly wasn't doing anything to fight the wrinkles that gave her face character and authority. I suspect she actually was close to sixty-five. What a beauty; it was all I could do to mind my manners and not express my admiration for this stranger!

After years of experience, I know that this woman was not cutting such a fine figure because of good genes, cosmetic surgery or any other "cheat" that

Victims believe separates the slender and overweight. This woman had taken good care of her body through exercise. Whatever her method, it was working beautifully, and I suspect it will for many years to come.

Your Method: Know the Benefits

The key to beginning a healthy new exercise regimen is being honest about what you like to do and what you don't. If you think that a gym membership or a personal trainer is essential but hate the way gyms smell and feel shy around people, chances are you're never going to get started. If you, like the majority of people in Western cultures, are pretty much inactive, you should start thinking outside the box. If you're a Victim who reflexively says "I can't" when the subject of exercise is exercised, you'll need to get creative. But make no mistake: you CAN exercise, vigorously, no matter what your situation might be.

Of course, just as it was when you determined to change your diet, you want to ramp up slowly to a new life of regular exercise. It made no sense to slash seven hundred calories from your diet on day one, and it also is unwise to start training vigorously for a triathlon if you haven't had any aerobic workouts in years. You want your doctor's OK and plan of action before you attempt to climb mountains (yes, please take that literally).

But then you're going to want a little spirit of adventure. If you're ready to exercise, it's also a great time to commit to learning or relearning a sport you enjoy. The best exercise efforts are those that don't feel like chores. If you enjoy a game of tennis and have a partner you're longing to beat handily, a workout on the court isn't going to feel like labor; it will pass before you know it and probably before you want it to end.

Take time to imagine the type of movement that will feel joyous. Dancing? Ultimate Frisbee? Cross-country skiing? Each is a terrific way to burn the calories and elevate your heart rate. Whether you like to compete against others or set private goals, there is activity that's ideal for you.

I'm willing to work with you even if you find all sports boring and believe any time spent exercising for exercise's sake is wasted time. Well then, what about vacuuming your house? Double benefit: clean house and exercise. If you vacuum on high intensity, it's a workout. I mean, it really is!

Remember that whatever you do—even sleeping—calories are burning. If you are an exercise foe and are determined to be useful every hour of the day, then clean like you never have before: floors (mop them, too), dusting, scrubbing. Clean out the closets. Throw out the trash. But get it done in record time. Move quickly. If you are such an efficiency maven, then move, move, move. Scrub the kitchen surfaces harder. Work up a sweat!

Are you proud of your garden? Well, the weeds are sprouting as we speak. Turn the soil, drag over the bags of fertilizer and put some effort into your landscaping. Do it faster than usual. Maintain your speed, unless you're increasing it.

You should see a basic principle here. Many activities that you currently enjoy or complete out of necessity are opportunities to burn fuel. If exercise is slowly making its way back into your routine, concentrate on giving more effort in the things that come naturally. If you are a new mother taking out the stroller, try doubling your usual pace (although to turn this into an aerobic exercise you'll need to outfit your baby with a harness and a crash helmet. Either that, or invest in a jogging stroller). Make sure you're moving quickly at least three times a week. With these building blocks in place, you'll soon be ready to try a real workout.

And if you like the convenience and bustle of a gym, take advantage of all it offers. Ask the staff what classes are best for burning calories. Explain that you're intent on increasing your metabolic rate and listen to their suggestions. They'll be happy to help. Yet again, you can manage instant gratification and a long-term investment.

Run, Lindsay, Run

Factors such as your physical health and chronic pain also will affect your exercise choices and their intensity. And of course, the more you weigh, the more calories you'll burn during any activity. Someone who weighs 200 pounds will burn more than a 175-pound companion if she is exercising at the same level of intensity, since there's 25 extra pounds to pull through every motion.

For the sake of simplicity, I'm going to introduce you to "Lindsay," who weighs 150 pounds. She wants to lose 30 of them, which will put her back at the healthy weight she enjoyed before her babies were born.

The list that follows will show you how many calories Lindsay can expect to burn during thirty minutes of various activities. Some of these are aerobic exercises (running, for instance); others are not (light yoga). But notice that many of less-intensive activities could easily become aerobic just by stepping up the pace and pushing a little harder. Remember, personal trainers and gym owners might tell you it's their way or no way at all, but you shouldn't believe them. Here are just a few of the countless options[3] Lindsay can employ to lose weight:

Activity	Calories Burned (1/2 hour)
Gardening	117
Walking, level surface	146
Walking briskly	221
Walking uphill, carrying 10–20 lbs.	248
Running, 12-minute mile	282
8.5-minute mile	374
6.5-minute mile	435
Swimming freestyle, light	197
Swimming freestyle, vigorous	333
Dancing, general	265
Dancing, aerobic long step	340
Hiking (uphill, carrying 10–20 lbs.)	248
Cross-country skiing	340
Tai Chi	102
Martial arts	265
Bicycling, 11–15 mph	272
Bicycling, 16–19 mph	408
Bicycling, 20+ mph	537
Squash	408

---

3 Source: Every Day Health calorie counter.

Soccer	289
Ice skating	238
Volleyball	136
Yoga, light	85
Yoga, vigorous	136
Vacuuming	112
Shoveling snow	218
Mowing lawn (power mower)	163
Cleaning, light	85
Cleaning, vigorous	113
Cooking	68

I hope you paid particular attention to the figures on walking, running, and yoga; they should demonstrate, loud and clear, how exercise keeps delivering returns once you've become accustomed to it. Even walking can get intensive in a hurry. And there's plenty of competition to be had even if you're walking alone. Buy a stopwatch and time your new morning walk. On the second morning, try to eclipse your first time, even if by a single second. You can have plenty of fun just trying to best yourself.

Joint Problems? Don't Despair

It's true the joints of people who played high-impact, competitive sports can tell some sad stories. The same is often true of people who have carried extra weight for a long time. Joint pain is part of daily life for many of us, and it does have an effect on what exercise regimen will work best.

If your knees are balky, running is not going to be a great choice. But swimming freestyle in the local pool can be wonderful aerobic exercise because water doesn't resist your movements like the hard ground beneath a running shoe. Rowing machines, elliptical trainers, and weight-training machines are other popular choices with people who complain of joint aches and stiffness.

If you have problems with your joints, you might have to be a little more inventive, and it may help you to consult with a trainer or your physician about what exercises you should consider. What you don't want is for the negative Victim-ese voice to start arguing that it's impossible for you to train. It's not impossible. If you start slowly and do some research, you can find exercises that will be easy on your soft points while making all the others more solid.

Sex, Sex, Sex. And More Sex.

Anyone who has spent time flipping through a glossy magazine has probably read about the benefits of regular sexual activity. The fact is that this isn't just a bunch of wishful thinking or gossip. Ideally, your *Yes, You Can* journey will include plenty of intimate recreation; it's an integral part of the physical package and a key to your self-esteem.

You might want to laugh at the notion of sex as part of your workout regimen, but those who enjoy it regularly have the last (and best) laugh. Lindsay can burn around 85 calories for every half hour she spends having sex. (She can burn almost as much by giving her partner a massage; how's that for mutual benefits?) If she pulls that off three times a week, she's accounting for around 250 calories, no small change if you take the long view. But that's just the surface of the physical and emotional benefits sex brings to life.

Women strengthen their pelvic floor muscles through regular sex; that's good news at any stage of life, and particular so when you're getting ready for a birth. Regular sex is a natural combatant of depression, and since this pleasure releases oxytocin, it also fights the blues by encouraging better sleep. By now you know how these benefits can reinforce each other: More sleep and better moods mean more energy, which makes more activity likely. More activity means weight loss, and there we are, back at the central purpose of this book.

Research also indicates that sex aides the release of antibodies, which combat illness in the here and now. Regular ejaculation (twenty times a month or more) may decrease a man's risk of prostate cancer at any age. And while we've all heard the stories of old fellows dropping dead during the act, the evidence suggests that men's risk of heart attack actually decreases if they remain sexually active. Orgasms are brief but intense bursts of energy that put the body into a high alert for a few seconds. They're like little fire drills for the heart, and they help keep that most essential muscle vibrant and responsive.

The act of making love, massaging a partner, and spending time in a sexual dance also has benefits to your health and looks. It acts like a lymphatic drainage massage and gets rids of unwanted fluids. You can lose one size after just one act of making love! Lymphatic drainage through professional massage is now being marketed heavily. Go see a professional if you want; appreciating and being appreciated will bring many of the same results.

There is no elixir that will provide eternal life; all we have are various means of counteracting the aging process. Well, it turns out that sex "keeps you young" for physical reasons, not just emotional ones! Testosterone levels in men naturally decrease with age, but regular sex encourages the production of more testosterone. Keeping busy in your bedroom (or wherever the mood strikes) will never stop time, but it just might slow it down.

The sex benefit that is most important might be the one you can't measure with a formula or statistic. But it's hard to keep good women and men down when they feel good about themselves and comfortable in their own skin. Sex at its best is an affirmation of your beauty and worth. A person who makes love regularly will find the old negative images of his or her body and self become wispier, ever easier to rip apart. When another person appreciates you and, most importantly, when *you* appreciate the sensations your body delivers, it's hard to fall back into destructive or indifferent habits.

Put it this way: I said in chapter one that by letter Z you would be treating your body like a temple. Well, what's a temple for? Go celebrate in it!

Youth Springs Eternal

Victim thinking has stalled many people when they attempted exercise, because there is one factor they believe they can never overcome, a factor that surely will get them in the end: their age.

There just isn't any point, some people have told me. Exercise is for young people, and they wasted their youth by being inactive and eating poorly. The road back to health will be too long, and even if they walk the entire length, what will they have to look forward to? The clock is ticking. They're middle aged already, or even older.

These people help me see that my job is also an A-to-Z process. I don't expect them to snap out of that terrible mind-set in a day. But during every hour I spend with them, I look for ways to demonstrate that I disagree with every single one of their assumptions and conclusions.

They assume they are no longer young. But really, what does "young" actually mean? Yes, eventually the cells of your body will display evidence that they've been working hard for many years. But what does youth really mean in the course of a lifetime?

Many of my clients arrived at my door when they were in their late forties or fifties. The weight problems were undeniable, but there were many positives in the lives of these people. They'd been working hard for years. Their children were either grown or getting ready to begin their own lives. They had wriggled out from underneath many of their toughest financial obligations. Although overweight, they still enjoyed reasonably good health.

Well, I would ask them, what do you have to look forward to?

A great deal as it turned out. Many discovered that the weight-loss process reconnected them with vigor they thought they'd left behind in their twenties. As they became more active and realized their bodies would respond when asked to push harder, they experienced physical joy again. Bombarded with endorphins and pride in their new shapes, they started to wonder what else might be possible.

They would begin to see the freedom they had won by weathering those difficult years. Little by little, the next twenty or thirty years began to appear as an astonishing land of opportunity. There were trips they could take, skills to learn, new degrees to study for, a life partner to get to know all over again. Sometimes there were new partners and friends to meet.

Once they caught a glimpse of all that possibility, their will to exercise often received a shot of adrenaline. Their nutritional IQs began to soar. Suddenly there was newfound purpose to their weight-loss goals. They saw that they were shedding more than extra flesh; they were shedding old routines and negative thinking that had sapped them of initiative and enthusiasm for so long.

No weight-loss program is magic. There are no wands you can wave that will instantaneously deliver a slim figure and brighter outlook on life. But I believe that taking charge of your life, your food, and your body certainly can transport you to a place you might only have dreamed about. It might be a place you once were and thought you could never find again.

You won't find that place in a day or a month, but every day you will see progress. You will realize it by degrees. With an open (and more oxygenated) mind, you'll discover that exercise isn't just for young, pretty people. It's for everyone, and with some concentrated effort, you'll find that motivation to get physical will come as naturally as thinking.

Summary

- *Moving is as necessary in 2013 as it was in 2013 BC.*

- *Extra activity isn't enough unless some of it is aerobic.*

- *Exercise delivers short- and long-term goals, much like putting money in the bank.*

- *Find an exercise that is enjoyable and that allows you to step up the pace gradually.*

- *You should count up the calories your favorite exercise requires*

- *The benefits of an active sex life go far beyond immediate pleasure.*

- *Exercise should never be wasted on the young.*

Chapter Eleven

TRAINING FOR LIFE

Enjoying the Z

Congratulations! You're here. You've crossed the finish line. Now's the time to feel good about yourself and all of the work you've put into achieving your ideal body.

Not yet? You still have another five pounds to lose? I still want you to celebrate. If you're closing in on the last five pounds, or even ten, you've made enormous changes in your life and achieved intermittent goals you probably thought were impossible when you began your journey.

You've changed deeply ingrained habits to reveal a better version of yourself. You've defeated one of the modern world's nastiest demons, a compulsive desire to overeat. You've become a Decision Maker and renounced victimhood. It's amazing.

And you've stopped demonizing food. You've learned how to balance six days of healthy eating against a weekly indulgence in your desire for chocolate, burgers and fries, whatever you once considered a "forbidden" food. There are no forbidden foods for you anymore. You know when to enjoy every food, and how often.

It's totally subjective, but many people would argue that it's easier to accumulate wealth than it is to shed weight and maintain your figure. Think about it for a moment. If you make some solid, early choices—a good career, investing in a varied portfolio, learning to budget—you will, over time, start to make money, which then makes more money, often by itself. If you figure out where to put your money it will multiply; if you learn who the best financial advisors are, you can delegate a great deal of your wealth-building activity.

But no one else can make all the diet choices that you make. No one can keep your portions under control but you. No one else can stop you from sinking your diet in a bakery or a fast-food drive-through. You can't be abducted, smuggled into a gym, and forced to exercise. And certainly no one else in the world can pinpoint your emotional eating triggers and learn how to get around them.

You've beaten long odds, just by assembling a long list of small challenges and meeting them day by day.

I lift my glass in a toast to you. I know how you feel; it is so empowering to take control of your weight. You may be starting to believe you can achieve many other goals in your life.

And guess what? You can.

You've lost weight, and with this book by your side and a high nutritional IQ, you know you can keep the weight off.

Well then. What else can you do?

Life after Success

I do have a few words of caution (don't worry, I won't spoil the party). There always will remain the possibility that you'll stop listening to your body. Hitting an established weight-loss goal prompts many people to declare that that's it, they're finished, and at once begin ignoring the new, healthy diet and approach to life they worked so hard to build.

You may see your victory as the end of the story, but it isn't. If you don't backslide, you won't have to work as hard as you did in the beginning, when you battled intense sugar cravings and every bit of exercise felt like torture; but you still have to work. Maintaining your body is a process that never ends, and your planning must remain careful and well thought out as you age.

Always listen to what your body needs and how it feels. Trust me: if you listen, it will answer. It will accept some changes. If your free meal has been Sunday lunch, but lately you fancy a high-caloric meal on Tuesdays, just make the change. If you feel you need to stop exercising for a couple of weeks because your favorite show is on in the evenings, by all means stop exercising. Everyone needs a vacation now and again.

There are a few rules that will never cease to apply. You worked hard to figure them out and become used to them. Now that you're at the goalpost, don't scrub them from your mental and muscle memory. Recite them, instead, every now and then as you maintain your beautiful body:

* Eat when you're hungry and stop when you're full.
* Know the calories of the foods that you're consuming,
* Eat clean foods.
* Avoid sugar as much as you can, especially the hidden and refined sugars.
* Be mindful of portion sizes.
* Eat breakfast.
* Drink plenty of water.
* Be active day by day, and raise your metabolic rate, through vigorous exercise, several times a week.
* Once a week, have a free meal; it is a must!

Maintaining your ideal body should be an enjoyable task. But life is tricky, and even the most diligent weight-control experts can find themselves, without warning, back in the middle of the alphabet. If it happens don't despair. That's life. Hopefully you won't shy from the work that will be required to reestablish your positive standard for weight and fitness. And you won't hate yourself for breaking a strong routine. We're human beings after all, not robots; we like our habits, but we're a quirky species, and sometimes we stray from the established path. When it comes to weight loss, you know the way back. You've been on it. You'll return to it.

Achieving New Goals

Now, back to the celebration. When you look in the mirror, a Decision Maker is looking back at you. The Victim you may have been is long gone; the Advice Asker is finally satisfied and committed to a path. People ask *you* for advice now about how to achieve their goals. You have something that others don't: determination and a clear plan of action.

Could now be the time to take what you've learned during your weight-loss journey and apply it to all the other areas in your life?

Maybe you want to leave an unsatisfying career and start your own business. Maybe you want improved relationships with the people you love. Maybe you wish to master a skill you've always admired, but have never had the courage to try.

Whatever it is, you can do it. You can do *anything*. You can use the same principles and methods you used to achieve your weight loss to solve any problem.

Let's have a play and imagine that you're ready to change jobs or begin a new career. Thinking back on the chapters of your book, how might you go about it?

* You won't make announcements: "Oh, on Monday I'm going to quit my job, get another one right away, and also break up with my boyfriend because he doesn't support me. By spring I will feng shui my life."

You know better than that. These pronouncements are unrealistic (by *Monday*?) and even if you haven't complained to your friends about your job before this, they'll think you're crazy. You know it's not wise to broadcast your intentions and set yourself up for failure, sabotage, and disappointment.

Instead, you'll take a good, long, quiet look at your situation, do some research, and then put your newfound confidence to work while you establish a game plan for change.

* Little steps count: Changing a job requires due diligence. You'll update your resume, survey the job market, network, and look into the training you might need to get current in your field. You'll do the little things that distinguish a focused, purposeful job search from a frantic, haphazard one. You'll

take control, and soon enough, control is what you'll project. And just maybe you'll realize the job you have now is not so bad at all.

* Sabotage: You are very cautious around family and friends who have a history of undermining your attempts to change. They aren't evil, and it probably isn't necessary that you avoid them altogether. But you keep in mind that they're probably quite scared of change themselves, and you need the presence of mind to disregard what they have to say about your career and aspirations.

Are you staying in your job because your friends and family convinced you that you are lucky to have it and that it is impossible to land great jobs in the current economy? Are they successful themselves?

One of my friends used to say, "A time of crisis is when you make more money and find better jobs because people are too scared to make changes, which means more opportunities for risk takers/decision makers."

* Controlling the internal dialogue: Remember when you used to eat out of habit or to fill an emotional hole? Maybe you are staying in your job out of habit; perhaps having a bad job and being unhappy is part of an old story you've been telling for years. Think carefully about whether or not this story really is true. Imagine having a new job and how success would make you feel. Keep imagining; you're rehearsing a new story.

Start to plan how to get a new job and fight your emotional habits, applying the same technique you used to fight emotional eating. Get busy. Talk to recruiters, or make connections in the field you love. Learn how people are making opportunity work for them. Get involved. Don't spend your nights whining (silently or otherwise) about how frustrating your current situation is. Change your state of mind. It will be gradual, but you know that the accumulation of small steps most certainly can complete this journey.

* Green, Yellow, and Red zones: As with weight loss, there are safe behaviors, risky ones, and some plainly outrageous options that you shouldn't even consider. Just flat out quitting your job before you know where the next paycheck is coming from is a Red zone impulse. Don't waste time applying for jobs that you aren't qualified for. Yellow zone behaviors include making inquiries, getting your name out in certain circles, perhaps volunteering to do work that might be a stretch for you but that will provide invaluable

experience. Green zone activities are fact-finding, conducting interviews, and learning everything you can about where you want to be and the job you aspire to attain.

Stay away from the outrageous Red options and mix it up between the safety of the Green and the riskier but potentially valuable action of the Yellow.

* Daily check-in and assessment (without being obsessed): While looking for a new position or a better career, you should be accountable to yourself every day. When you lost weight, you stepped on the scale every morning. As a job hunter, every night ask yourself what you did to move toward your goal. Some days will be better than others, but you'll look to your common denominator of progress and know if you're really moving forward or spinning your wheels.

* Keep in fighting trim: In this case, it's not move, move, move but think, think, and think some more. Your mind should be active no matter what you're doing. Cut back on drinking, TV, and other passive activities and make sure you're keeping current with ideas. Retain interest in life outside of your career. Ask big questions. Schedule productive downtime and exercise (yes, it helps in these situations, too).

A Program for Life: Having It All?

It's all up to you, really. You and nobody else, my dear Decision Maker.

You can decide how you want your life to look, just as you decided how you wanted your body to look and feel when you began your weight-loss journey.

But now, successful in one endeavor, can you expand your vision? Can you really have it all?

That's another popular phrase, one so popular that it has become almost meaningless. But it shouldn't be. You should undertake a good, healthy investigation of that phrase and the concepts behind it.

"Having it all" is totally subjective, but society at large has its own, powerful opinion. Most of us in the Western world probably imagine "perfect" happiness is impossible without plenty of money. And a blissful marriage with smart, beautiful children. And a fulfilling career.

Hmmm.

If you've been a Victim or Advice Asker, it's probably quite easy to assume that that gauzy definition of happiness is synonymous with having it all. Pretty much anything else would fall short.

Our society tells us a lot about what we *think* we should value. But tuning out your own ideas in favor of society's collective is a reactive mindset, not a natural one. Who really lives in that world of "perfect" happiness? Probably no one.

To know what it really means to have it all, you need yet again to stop, listen, and think about yourself. The answer is in *there*, not out here.

It's entirely possible that your true aspiration really is for wealth, beauty, and romance rolled into one fashionable package. But it's also possible that true fulfillment could mean leaving a lucrative but crazy job and moving to the countryside to grow vegetables and sell them at the farmer's market. Maybe you witnessed animal cruelty as a child and happiness entails adopting forsaken dogs. Perhaps it's dependent on you deciding once and for all that having children is not a necessity. Maybe it means returning to medical school or working for the Salvation Army.

Who defines your happiness? You do.

How do you attain it?

That requires a lot of honesty, and discipline, too. But of course, you know discipline now; you wouldn't have lost weight if you couldn't keep to a regimen. And now that you know how to lose weight and achieve the body of your dreams, you have the tools to achieve all of your goals, whether you yet believe it or not. Losing weight is about visualizing a goal—a finish line—and slowly, mindfully, making your way toward it, even when there are setbacks along the way. It's about staying focused on what's important to you.

So let's work on honesty. Take the time to let your inner self show up in the mirror and in your thoughts.

Make another list. Visualize all of your goals and write them down. Then, slowly, like a turtle, start walking toward them.

You will recognize easily the saboteurs and avoid emotional tantrums. You will be your first cheerleader, and your internal dialogue will be the essential tool for achieving your goals.

As you did when you learned to evaluate hunger, you should regularly ask yourself, "Do I really want this? Does this goal really mean something to me? Will it improve my quality of life? Do I want it just because others want it or tell me that I should?"

Looking into yourself means stripping away layers of expectation. It's hard to dig down to the honest core of yourself. But make no mistake: trying to achieve what others told you to achieve is another form of sabotage. It's to be a follower. A Decision Maker sets an original course.

You may discover that "having it all" may not include marriage or great riches. So what? There are plenty of other people in the world who can manage those aspirations. Your ambition is unique.

You want to write a novel? You can. The hardest part is starting, but you can do it. Take a pen and start writing, ignoring the inner sabotaging voice that says you're wasting your time. If the voice is loud, just tell it to shut up and keep writing. Like with weight loss, don't make pronouncements to everyone about how you're writing a novel. Just write it and tell people about it when you've completed it. As with weight loss, there will be moments when you feel hopeless or stuck; just push through those moments and keep going. One day you'll look up and realize that you've achieved your goal of completing a novel. Then you can set new goals: write a second, revise the first, create a Web platform for the book, get it published, or publish it yourself. Don't rest on that accomplishment; find the letter A once more and begin a new journey.

You want to buy a house? Well then, start saving your pennies and improving your credit rating. Learn everything you can about real estate, and quietly, without making waves, look for something that you can afford. Educate yourself about loans for homeowners. Explore different neighborhoods, and ask your homeowner friends for tips. As with weight loss, it won't happen unless you try to make it happen. It will take some time, but one day you'll be moving into the dream house that you bought.

It's easy to slip into victimhood when it you begin to chase your goals in earnest. You may think, "Yes, I'm no longer overweight and I've achieved the body that I want, but I can't quit my job and start my own business. That's too hard."

Ridiculous. You can. I'm not encouraging anyone to impulsively quit a job, but if you have a great idea for a business, why not start working toward making it real? This will mean raising your IQ (as you did with nutrition) about your field of interest and taking the steps to understand what a real, concentrated effort in business will look like. But why can't you do it? What, really, is the difference between you, the weight loser, and you, the entrepreneur?

Is there a difference?

You can also apply your weight-loss tools to your relationships. Maybe you'd like to improve your family life. You can stage a detoxification by discontinuing the behaviors that have driven you apart from your loved ones. You can make a pledge to open communication back up, one small step at a time. You can look long and hard at the history you and your spouse share, and try to reconnect outside the ruts of routine and kneejerk responses. If you are the only one who wants to change, you can take steps—through therapy, friends, and work channels—to start imagining a new life on your own.

Goal achievement breeds deep satisfaction in all of us. It makes us happy. The happiness will linger if, after a period of celebration, a new goal is envisioned and a plan is implemented. That's what life is about: Working toward something, always moving forward.

I hope that by completing your weight-loss journey, you have realized the power that you have inside of you to change, not just your body and your health, but your life.

Can you really achieve what you want? Of course, yes, you can.

The journey has already begun. And remember: Be careful what you wish for. You could get it.

Summary

- Maintaining your ideal body is a lifelong journey.

- As you continue on your journey, remember the tools you learned as you achieved your weight-loss goals.

- The strategies you used to lose weight can be applied to all areas of your life to achieve what you want.

BIBLIOGRAPHY

Books

Brand-Miller, Jennie, et al. *The New Glucose Revolution* (Marlowe, 2003).

Pennington, Jean A. T., and Judith S. Spungen. *Bowes and Church's Food Values of Portions Commonly Used,* 19th ed. (Lippincott Williams & Wilkins 2010).

Wansink, Brian. *Mindless Eating* (Bantam, 2006).

Articles

Avena, Nicole M., Pedro Rada, and Bartley G. Hoebel. "Evidence for Sugar Addiction: Behavioral and Neurochemical Effects of Intermittent, Excessive Sugar Intake." *Neuroscience Biobehavioral Review* 32(1) (2008): 20–39.

Johnson, Paul M., Paul J. Kenny. "Dopamine D2 Receptors in Addiction-Like Reward Dysfunction and Compulsive Eating in Obese Rats." *Nature Neuroscience* 13(5) (2010): 635.

Neumark-Sztainer, D., K. W. Bauer, S. Friend, P. J. Hannan, M. Story, J. M. Berge. "Family Weight Talk and Dieting: How Much Do They Matter for Body Dissatisfaction and Disordered Eating Behaviors in Adolescent Girls?" *Journal of Adolescent Health* 47(3) (September 2010): 270–76.

Walsh, Jean A., et al. "Caloric Sweetener Consumption and Dyslipidemia among US Adults." *JAMA.* 303(15) (2010): 1490-97.

Useful Web sites

BMI charts: www.nhlbi.nih.gov/guidelines/obesity/bmi_tbl.htm

BMR formulas: www.bmi-calculator.net/bmr-calculator/
harris-benedict-equation

Diet soda intake: http://www.sciencedaily.com/releases/2011/06/110627183944.htm

Dietary reference intakes: http://fnic.nal.usda.gov/nal_display/index.php?info_
center=4&tax_level=3&tax_subject=256&topic_id=1342&level3_id=5140

General nutrition info:

www.nutrition.gov

www.cdc.gov/nutrition/everyone/resources/index.html

http://fnic.nal.usda.gov/nal_display/index.

php?info_center=4&tax_level=1&tax_subject=279

www.eufic.org/index/en

Metabolic syndrome: www.nhlbi.nih.gov/guidelines/cholesterol/index.htm

National Weight Control Registry: www.nwcr.ws

Pesticides in food: Environmental Working Group: www.ewg.org

Portion sizes: http://img.webmd.com/dtmcms/live/webmd/consumer_assets/
site_images/media/pdf/diet/portion-control-guide.pdf

Sugar in the diet: www.cspinet.org

WHR: National Heart, Lung, and Blood Institute, National Institutes of
Health. *The Practical Guide: Identification, Evaluation, and Treatment of Overweight and Obesity in Adults* (NIH Publication No. 00-4084). Available online:
http://www.nhlbi.nih.gov/guidelines/obesity/prctgd_c.pdf.